Principles of Pediatric Neurosurgery

Series Editor: Anthony J. Raimondi

Principles of Pediatric Neurosurgery

Head Injuries in the Newborn and Infant

The Pediatric Spine I: Development and Dysraphic State
The Pediatric Spine II: Developmental Anomalies
The Pediatric Spine III: Cysts, Tumors, and Infections

*Edited by Anthony J. Raimondi, Maurice Choux,
and Concezio Di Rocco*

The Pediatric Spine III
Cysts, Tumors, and Infections

Edited by Anthony J. Raimondi,
Maurice Choux, and Concezio Di Rocco

With 87 Figures

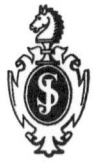

Springer Verlag
New York Berlin Heidelberg
London Paris Tokyo

ANTHONY J. RAIMONDI, 37020 Gargagnago (Verona), Italy

MAURICE CHOUX, M.D., Hôpital des Enfants de la Timone, Rue Saint Pierre, 13005 Marseille, France

CONCEZIO DI ROCCO, M.D., Istituto di Neurochirurgia, Università Cattolica del Sacro Cuore, Largo Gemelli 8, 00168 Rome, Italy

Library of Congress Cataloging-in-Publication Data
The pediatric spine.
    (Principles of pediatric neurosurgery)
    Includes bibliographies and index.
    Contents: 1. Development and the dysraphic
state— — 3. Cysts, tumors, and infections.
    1. Spine—Diseases. 2. Spine—Abnormalities.
3. Spine—Surgery. 4. Pediatric neurology. I. Raimondi,
Anthony J., 1928–   . II. Choux, M. (Maurice)
III. Di Rocco, C. (Concezio) IV. Series. [DNLM:
1. Spinal Diseases—in infancy and childhood. 2. Spine—
growth & development. WE 725 P3711]
RD768.P36 1989   618.92'73   88-24822

© 1989 by Springer-Verlag New York Inc.
Softcover reprint of the hardcover 1st edition 1989

Typeset by David E. Seham Associates, Inc., Metuchen, New Jersey.

9 8 7 6 5 4 3 2 1

ISBN-13:978-1-4613-8809-8   e-ISBN-13:978-1-4613-8807-4
DOI: 10.1007/978-1-4613-8807-4

Series Preface

It is estimated that the functionally significant body of knowledge for a given medical specialty changes radically every 8 years. New specialties and "sub-specialization" are occurring at approximately an equal rate. Historically, established journals have not been able either to absorb this increase in publishable material or to extend their readership to the new specialists. International and national meetings, symposia and seminars, workshops and newsletters successfully bring to the attention of physicians within developing specialties what is occurring, but generally only in demonstration form without providing historical perspective, pathoanatomical correlates, or extensive discussion. Page and time limitations oblige the authors to present only the essence of their material.

Pediatric neurosurgery is an example of a specialty that has developed during the past 15 years. Over this period, neurosurgeons have obtained special training in pediatric neurosurgery, and then dedicated themselves primarily to its practice. Centers, Chairs, and educational programs have been established as groups of neurosurgeons in different countries throughout the world organized themselves respectively into national and international societies for pediatric neurosurgery. These events were both preceded and followed by specialized courses, national and international journals, and ever-increasing clinical and investigative studies into all aspects of surgically treatable diseases of the child's nervous system.

Principles of Pediatric Neurosurgery is an ongoing series of publications, each dedicated exclusively to a particular subject, a subject which is currently timely either because of an extensive amount of work occurring in it, or because it has been neglected. The two first subjects, "Head Injuries in the Newborn and Infant" and "The Pediatric Spine," are expressive of those extremes.

Volumes will be published continuously, as the subjects are dealt with, rather than on an annual basis, since our goal is to make this information available to the specialist when it is new and informative. If a volume becomes obsolete because of newer methods of treatment and concepts, we shall publish a new edition.

The chapters are selected and arranged to provide the reader, in each instance, with embryological, developmental, epidemiological, clinical, therapeutic, and psychosocial aspects of each subject, thus permitting each specialist to learn what is current in his field and to familiarize himself with sister fields of the same subject. Each chapter is organized along classical lines, progressing from introduction through symptoms and treatment, to prognosis, for clinical material; and introduction through history and data, to results and discussion, for experimental material.

Contents

Contributors

ADELOLA ADELOYE
Department of Surgery, University College Hospital, University of
Ibadan, Ibadan, Nigeria

ANTONELLO CEDDIA
Istituto di Neurochirurgia, Università Cattolica del Sacro Cuore, Rome,
Italy

CESARE COLOSIMO JR.
Istituto di Radiologia, Università Cattolica del Sacro Cuore, Rome,
Italy

CONCEZIO DI ROCCO
Istituto di Neurochirurgia, Università Cattolica del Sacro Cuore, Rome,
Italy

ALDO IANNELLI
Istituto di Neurochirurgia, Università Cattolica del Sacro Cuore, Rome,
Italy

GÉRARD MONFORT
Centre Hospitalier de la Timone, Hôpital des Enfants, Marseille,
France

SAMUEL NEFF
Department of Neurosurgery, New England Medical Center and Tufts
University School of Medicine, Boston, Massachusetts, USA

RAINER W. OBERBAUER
Neurosurgical Department, University of Graz, Graz, Austria

WARWICK J. PEACOCK
Division of Neurosurgery, The Center for the Health Sciences,
University of California at Los Angeles, Los Angeles, California, USA

ANTHONY J. RAIMONDI
Northwestern University Medical School, Chicago, Illinois, USA
(Emeritus) and Dipartimento di Neurochirurgia, Università degli Studi,
Verona, Italy

R. MICHAEL SCOTT
Childrens Hospital, Boston, Massachusetts, USA

JOAN L. VENES
Section of Neurosurgery, Department of Surgery, University of
Michigan, Ann Arbor, Michigan, USA

CHAPTER 1

Spinal Meningeal Malformations

Concezio Di Rocco, Antonello Ceddia,
and Cesare Colosimo Jr.

Introduction

Spinal meningeal malformations include idiopathic intraspinal arachnoid
cysts, paravertebral meningoceles, anterior sacral meningoceles, and perineurial cysts (Tarlov's cyst) (34). These malformations should be distinguished from acquired cysts of the meninges, which may develop after
trauma, laminectomy, or lumbar puncture. Cystic meningeal malformations
usually become symptomatic in children aged from 10 to 12 years, in ad-
olescence, and in adulthood.

Intraspinal Arachnoid Cysts

Idiopathic intraspinal arachnoid cysts originate from the arachnoid of the
spinal cord, which extends to the sheaths of the roots of the spinal nervus.
They may appear as an isolated cystic mass lesion, which does not communicate with the subarachnoid space or, more commonly, as an expanding diverticulum of the arachnoid, continuing into the subarachnoid
space through a relatively narrow neck (25). Intraspinal arachnoid cysts
may remain confined within the intradural space (intradural arachnoid
cysts) or may protrude into the extradural space through a dural defect
(extradural arachnoid cysts). These cysts rarely exhibit both intradural
and extradural components (8). According to some, they may develop
"interdurally," between the leaves of the dura (9), but this is difficult to
understand anatomically since there is only one layer of dura enveloping
the spinal arachnoid.

The pathogenesis of intraspinal arachnoid cysts has remained a subject
of continuous debate since first described by Schlesinger in 1898 (46).
Their frequent association with other congenital spinal anomalies (diastematomyelia, intervertebral fusion) and their occurrence in members of
the same family and in persons with Recklinghausen's disease constitute
the basis of all theories that postulate the congenital nature of these cysts.

So far, however, there has been no convincing explanation for all the different types of spinal arachnoid cysts. Some authors believe that intraspinal arachnoid cysts result from the widening of the septum posticum, which separates the dorsal spinal subarachnoid space at the midline in the cervical and thoracic areas (26,39). Such a pathogenetic interpretation would account for the frequent occurrence of congenital spinal arachnoid cysts in the cervical and dorsal spinal regions (in contrast with the acquired postinfective and posttraumatic cystic dilatations of the arachnoid, which prevail at the lumbar level). It does not explain, however, the pathogenesis of the cysts located anterior to the spinal cord or in the proximity of the spinal roots.

According to a second explanation, spinal arachnoid cysts represent herniation of the arachnoid membrane due to congenital defects of the dura mater (16). Obviously, this hypothesis does not explain the origin of cysts confined exclusively within the dural sac. A more unitary pathogenetic interpretation considers spinal arachnoid cysts the result of the abnormal arrangement of the trabeculae, which develop within the subarachnoid space during the early embryogenic period. Arachnoid diverticula would form and subsequently enlarge because of the pressure exerted by the cerebrospinal fluid (CSF) on these aberrantly proliferated and distributed trabeculae, probably through a valvular mechanism (4,53).

Intradural Cysts

These cysts are rare in children and usually are discovered in adulthood (25). Men and women are equally affected. In most patients these lesions are found at the dorsal level, posterior or lateroposterior to the spinal cord; however, cervical and lumbar locations have also been reported (36,38). Rarely do intradural arachnoid cysts develop anterior or anterolateral to the spinal cord (37). Intradural arachnoid cysts may occur as single, multisegmental or multiple dilatations of the arachnoid space. In particular, arachnoid cysts have been described in association with extradural and perineural cysts (41) or in patients with ankylosing spondylitis (20,33). Most of these lesions are relatively large, extending over several segments of the spine and exerting a compression on the spinal cord and surrounding CSF spaces. However, in spite of their dimensions, only in rare cases do these cysts provoke an anomaly of the statics of the spine. In children, however, an enlargement of the spinal canal can be observed (1,14,37).

Clinical manifestations may vary in different patients and, with time, in the same person. Indeed, clinical symptoms—local or radicular pain, dysesthesia, motor deficits, and bladder disturbances—evolve over a period of months or years, with transitory episodes of remission in some cases, which mimic demyelinating diseases (37,41). In other instances an exacerbation with changes in posture reflects fluctuations in volume of the cyst or a secondary stretching of the adjacent neural structures (4).

A plain X-ray film of the spine is rarely of any help (2) in diagnosing intradural cysts. In fact, most of these cysts described in the literature have been diagnosed with myelography, which may demonstrate the cyst directly if the contrast medium enters it. More frequently, the examination suggests the presence of an intradural mass lesion with or without a complete CSF block. In most cases opacification of the cyst is slight because of its usually narrow neck. This opacification occurs minutes or hours after the first series of myelographic films.

Computed tomography (CT), after intrathecal injection of contrast medium (so-called "myelo-CT"), may be regarded as the diagnostic method of choice because of its superior contrast resolution capabilities (Fig. 1.1). In some cases, however, the neuroradiological differential diagnosis between intradural spinal cysts and other cystic conditions may remain difficult; such is the case, for example, of the cystic dilatation of the dural sac accompanying maldevelopmental tumors in which the spinal cord may be extremely thinned (Fig. 1.2).

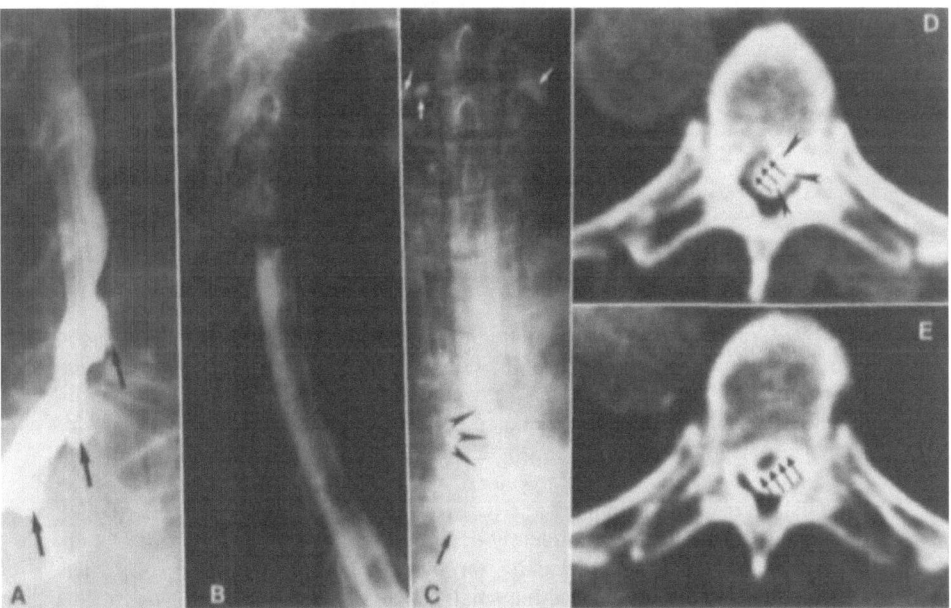

Figure 1.1. Intradural arachnoid cyst at T-5 level; multiple perineurial cyst of the lumbar, thoracic, and cervical root sleeves. A–C Myelography. Multiple perineurial cysts (*arrows*) of the lumbar, thoracic, and cervical root sleeves. At T-4 to T-5 level there is a right intradural hemispheric mass (*arrowheads*) resulting in a transitory block (**B**), **D,E** Myelo-CT (contiguous axial slices obtained one hour after myelogram). There is a densely opacificied lesion (*arrowheads*) occupying the spinal canal and displacing the flattened spinal cord controlaterally (*arrows*). At surgery, intradural arachnoid cyst was excised. Adjacent to cyst, there was a small angioma.

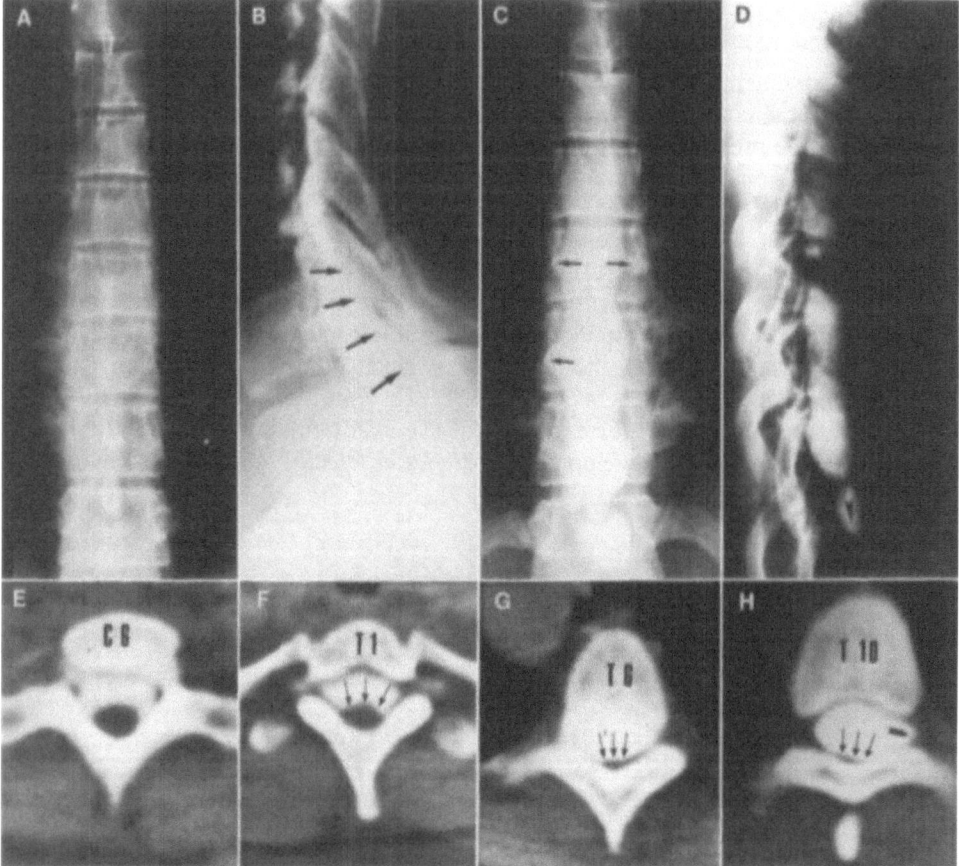

Figure 1.2. Cystic dilation of the subarachnoid space of the dorsal tract associated with maldevelopmental tumor of the cauda equina. **A** Anteroposterior (AP) film of the thoracic spine demonstrates an extreme thinning of the dorsal pedicles with widening of the interpediculate distance. **B** Laterocervical myelography reveals a normal situation up to C-5; from the C-5 level the subarachnoid space anterior to the spinal cord begins to enlarge (*arrows*) with progressive reduction of the sagittal diameter of the spinal cord. **C,D** From the cervicodorsal junction to T-9, the enlarged spinal canal is completely occupied by the enlarged, "cystic," subarachnoid space, which also herniates through the neuroforamina (*arrows*). The cystic dilatation ends caudally with a small saccular loculation (*arrowhead*). **F-H** Myelo-CT confirms the myelographic data and demonstrates that the spinal cord moves posteriorly and becomes progressively flattened from the lower cervical up to the upper thoracic level. Here the cord is reduced to an extremely thin layer (*arrows*). Note also herniation of the dural sac through the neuroforamen (*arrowhead*).

A remission of symptoms is achieved in the majority of patients after surgical excision of the cyst. The lesion appears as a traslucent, round, or oval cystic formation—a few centimeters in diameter—that fluctuates with respiratory movements. In less than a third of the cases, intradural arachnoid cysts assume a diverticular morphology. A relatively common operative finding is the presence of associated anomalous vessels on the dorsal aspect of the spinal cord (38) (Fig. 1.1). In a few cases the cystic lining is adherent to the spinal cord or nerve roots, thus preventing complete surgical removal (25). In such cases the shunting of the cyst into the peritoneal cavity has been recommended, especially when a radiological examination reveals the reaccumulation of fluid (6).

Extradural Cysts

These are fairly evenly distributed throughout all ages, with, however, a bimodal peak considerably higher in the 10- to 15-year-age group, and lesser in the 16- to 20-year age group. Cases occurring in young children, adults, and elderly patients have been described as well (44,55). Males are slightly more frequently affected than females. Although sporadic in most cases, extradural arachnoid cysts may occur in families with lymphedema (Milroy's disease) and distichiasis (double row of eyelashes) as an autosomal trait (7,43). Dumbbell extradural arachnoid cysts may also develop in the thoracic cavity, as a paraspinal mass, in subjects with Marfan's syndrome (8). In most cases these cysts appear as membranous diverticula connected by a narrow neck to a nerve root sleeve and are usually situated at the root entry into the spinal subarachnoid space. They are less commonly located on the posterior midline or in proximity to the point of fixation of the filum terminale. By taking into account this characteristic topography, a mechanical hypothesis has been propounded to explain the genesis of this type of cyst since extradural arachnoid cysts develop through areas of lower resistance of the dura mater (16). Indeed, the lateral meningoradicular junctions constitute a frequent site of abnormal arachnoid proliferation and cystic cavity formation (42). However, for some authors the extradural arachnoid cysts situated in the lumbar region and close to the attachment of the filum terminale could be likened to meningoceles and would thus originate from a defective closure of the posterior neuropore (23). The large majority of extradural arachnoid cysts are situated posterior or posterolateral to the dural sac, most frequently in the thoracic regions (11). Only rarely do these cysts lie anterior to the theca (37). In almost half the cases, they develop along the intervertebral foramina and eventually grow into paraspinal masses in the chest (8,30).

Progressive limb weakness, associated in some patients with low thoracic or abdominal pain, is the most common presenting complaint; bowel and bladder dysfunction have also been described, although less frequently than in cases of intradural cysts (10,11). In about a third of the cases the symptoms are intermittent, with periods of remission. It is worth noting that despite the frequent posterior location of these cysts, pain and sensorial disturbances are usually much less pronounced than the motor deficit. The frequent occurrence of vertebral deformities (kyphoscoliosis is found in about half the patients with a dorsal cyst) suggests that extradural arachnoid cysts may remain silent for a long time before diagnosis.

Most of the extradural arachnoid cysts communicate with the arachnoid space through a narrow pedicle. The ostium is typically situated at the cranial end of the cyst (34): In some patients it may act as a one-way valve because of the folding of the meninges (21), or it may eventually close, thus isolating the cyst from the subarachnoid space (28,51). In communicating cysts, three main mechanisms are thought to account for the enlargement of the lesion and for its compressive effect on the spinal cord. These are (a) a one-way valve causing an intermittent increase in pressure, (b) a hyperosmolar collection of fluid, and (c) the secretion of fluid by the cyst wall itself (in cases of isolated cysts) (44).

Radiological evaluation of the spine may show an enlargement of the spinal canal, erosion of the pedicles, and scalloping of the vertebral bodies, which suggest long-standing compression exerted by the lesion. Again, myelography, myelo-CT and MRI are the diagnostic methods of choice. The opacification of the cyst by intrathecal contrast medium is better demonstrated by means of late myelo-CT evaluation (from one to 24 hours after myelography) (Fig. 1.3). However, in most cases, especially in the extended ones, opacification is not observed (Fig. 1.4). In such a situation the diagnosis may be suggested by evidence of the long-standing compressive effect with relatively slight neurological symptoms, by the posterior extradural site of the mass lesion, and—above all—by the hypodense content (CSF-like) of the "tumor."

At surgery, extradural arachnoid cysts appear as relatively large lesions usually extending over two to six vertebral segments, with a thin, translucent wall. Epidural fat corresponding to the lesion is normally absent. The dural sac is usually displaced anteriorly or laterally as are the roots of the cauda equina in cases of sacral location. Complete excision of the cyst lining can usually be accomplished and should be regarded as the preferable way to treat the lesion, although an improvement in clinical conditions has been described following either the simple aspiration of the cyst or its subtotal resection. Rarely, the removal of the cyst may be complicated by adherence of its membrane to the posterior surface of the dura mater, or its extension into the neural foramina. With regard to intradural cysts, the benign nature of these lesions and their large size, which may require a wide exposure of the spinal canal during operative procedures, suggest the need to spare the posterior arch to prevent spine instability. This is accomplished by performing a spinal *laminotomy* rather than a *laminectomy,* especially in younger children or in patients presenting a kyphoscoliotic deformity (9,40).

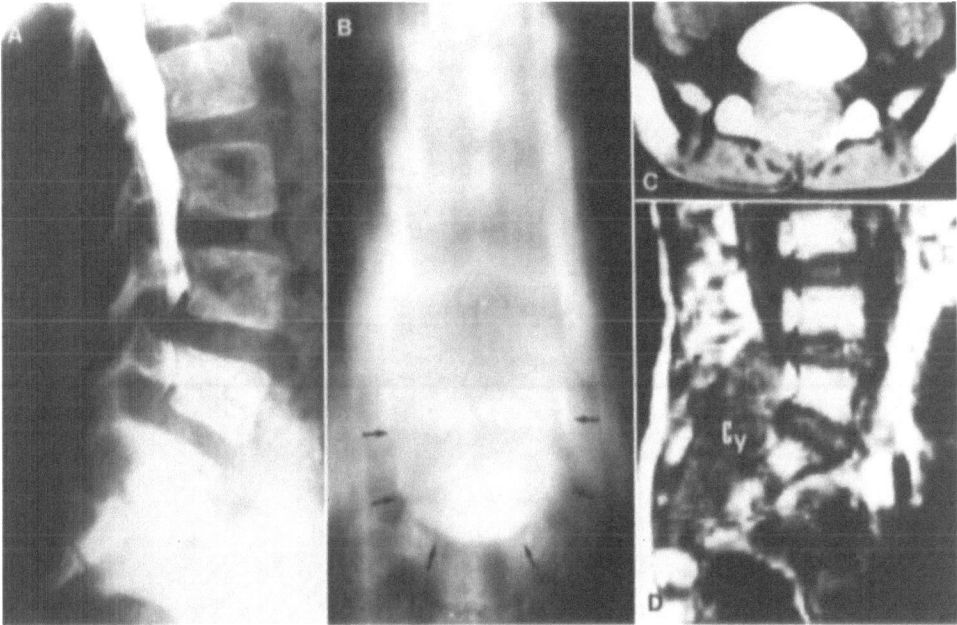

Figure 1.3. Large extradural posterior cyst at the lumbosacral junction. **A** Myelography shows a posterior extradural mass lesion flattening the dural sac. Note the enlargement of the sacral canal. **B** Myelotomography one hour after the introduction of contrast medium reveals subtle opacification of a "pouch" (*arrows*) in the most dependent part of the cystic lesion. **C** Late myelo-CT confirms opacification of the cyst. **D** At magnetic resonance imaging, MRI, (sagittal T-1-weighted image) the large ovoid cystic sac (Cy) exhibits an intensity slightly higher than the subarachnoid CSF. This finding results from the increased protein content in the cystic CSF (28).

Paravertebral Meningoceles

A CSF-filled protrusion of the dura and arachnoid may herniate out of the spine, anteriorly through a defect in the vertebral body or laterally through an enlarged neural foramen.

Anterior Sacral Meningoceles

These usually occur at the level of the sacrum and coccyx but can be found at any level. They are related to a congenital bone defect that allows the formation of a CSF-filled hernia sac in the pelvis. Associated anomalies include Marfan's syndrome, neurofibromatosis (Fig. 1.5), dermoids, lipomas, teratomas, imperforate anus, and duplication of the uterus, vagina,

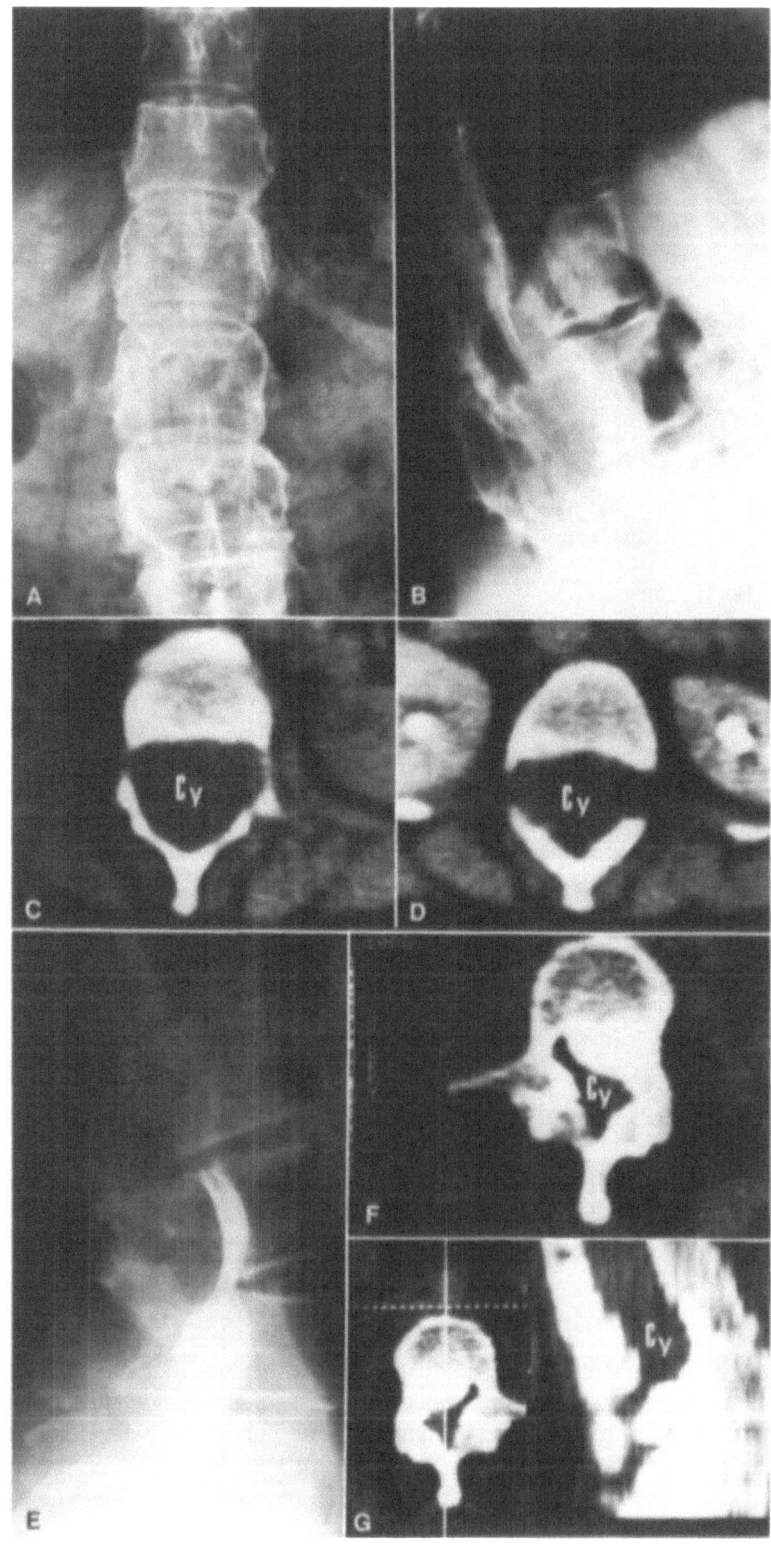

kidneys, and ureters (24,32,48,49). In adults this type of malformation is three times more common in women; in the pediatric population (27) it is equally distributed among the two sexes. This apparent difference is likely the result of frequent pelvic examinations in postmenarche women. Symptoms depend on visceral compression (urinary frequency and incontinence, unremitting constipation, low back or pelvic pain), on pressure exerted on adjacent nerve roots (sciatica, sphincter impairment, paresthesia, and, rarely, motor deficits of the lower limbs), and on intermittently increased intracranial pressure due to movement of the CSF from the herniated sac into the spinal subarachnoid space (48).

Radiological abnormalities in the sacral anterior meningoceles are commonly detected on x-ray films; these include enlargement of the sacral canal and scalloping and erosion of the sacral segments as well as the presence of a well-defined defect in the anterior wall of the sacral bone (22,48). The malformed sacrum often assumes the curvilinear appearance of a scimitar, which is a typical finding of the condition. The coccyx is often absent (48). The sac herniated within the pelvis may reach a considerable size. It is lined by a simple layer of squamous or columnar epithelium with mucus-laden cells (3), and it communicates with the spinal subarachnoid spaces through a usually narrow neck in the region of the anterior sacral defect.

Anterior sacral meningoceles can be either excised or ligated at the neck. However, ligation can be prevented in some patients by the presence of nerve roots and filum terminale passing through the neck into the hernia sac, or by the large size of the neck itself (15).

Anterior Thoracic Meningoceles

These develop in the mediastinum by protruding through a defect in the body of a thoracic vertebra. They are extremely rare (45).

Lateral Thoracic Meningoceles

These are found in the extrapleural posterolateral thoracic gutter and originate from a protrusion of the dura and arachnoid through an enlarged

---

Figure 1.4. Giant extradural cyst from L-3 to T-6. **A,B** Plain film reveals marked enlargement of the spinal canal with severe scalloping in the dorsolumbar junction. **C,D** Intravenous-enhanced CT does not show any increase in density of the liquid hypodense lesion (CY), which also herniates through the neuroforamina. **E** Myelography reveals an extradural mass lesion that displaces anteriorly and flattens the thecal sac, resulting in a complete block. **F,G** Myelo-CT with sagittal reformation (**G**) fails to show any detail of the cyst (Cy), which is posterior to the thecal sac.

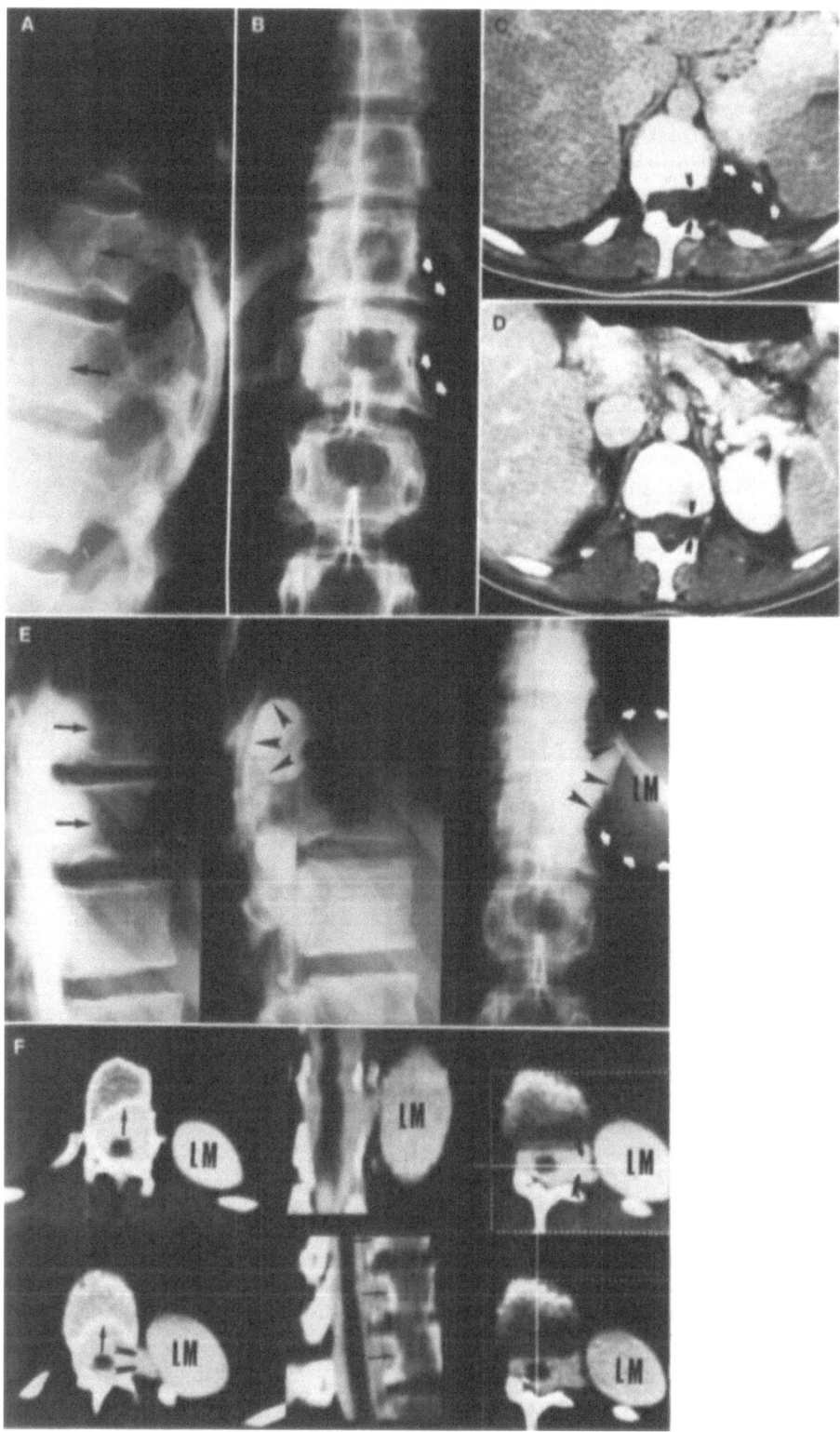

neural foramen, extending anteriorly through the adjacent intercostal space. The malformation is more commonly encountered in adults and in patients with neurofibromatosis (17). The right side is more frequently affected, although in a few patients the malformation can be bilateral (usually more extensive on the right side) or confined to the left side. The communication between the sac and the spinal subarachnoid space occurs more commonly at the level of only one intervertebral foramen, usually in the upper thoracic spine. Lateral thoracic meningoceles may remain silent for a long period of time or cause a mild neurological symptom, such as pain or vague sensory or motor deficits. In newborn, however, they may cause respiratory disturbances (5).

Scoliosis of the upper thorac spine (convex toward the meningocele) and kyphosis are the prominent radiological findings and are associated with an enlargement of the neural foramen, thinning of the pedicles and of the laminae, and scalloping of the vertebral bodies. The adjacent intercostal space may be widened and the margins of the ribs eroded (31,17) (Figs. 1.5 and 1.6).

At surgical exploration, the lesion may range from a very small sac to a mass occupying the entire hemithorax. Neural structures are absent. Complete excision may be difficult because of adherences to the parietal pleura and some other structures. Shunting of the lateral cerebral ventricles may succeed in determining the disappearance of the sac (31).

Lateral Lumbar Meningoceles

These develop within the lumbar subcutaneous tissue or in the retroperitoneal region through an enlargement of one or more neural foramina of the lumbar spine (18). The kidneys and ureters are the most commonly compressed structures; neurological signs are rare. Radiological abnormalities consist of the enlargement of the spinal canal and neural foramina, erosion of the posterior surface of the vertebral bodies, and thinning of the laminae.

◁——

Figure 1.5. A 25-year-old woman with known Recklinghausen's disease. A,B Lateral and AP films demonstrate severe scalloping of the posterior vertebral bodies T-11, T-12 (*arrows*) with deformity of the left lateral aspect of the T-12 and T-11 vertebrae (*white arrows*). C,D Intravenous-enhanced CT reveals a left hypodense liquid-containing paravertebral pouch (*arrows*) with intraspinal/intraforamina extension (*arrowheads*). E Myelography opacifies and outlines the anterior intravertebral meningoceles (*black arrows*), the foraminal pouch (*arrowheads*), and the large less-dense lateral meningocele pouch (LM, *white arrows*). F Myelo-CT (with coronal and sagittal reformatted images) confirms the myelographic data showing the intravertebral pouches (*black arrows*), the foraminal sac (*arrowhead*), the large lateral meningocele (LM), and the normal spinal cord.

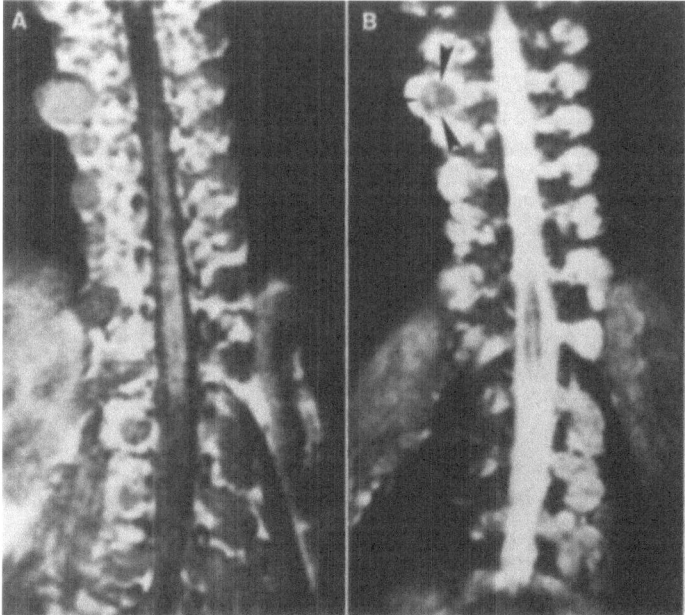

Figure 1.6. Diffuse dural ectasia in Recklinghausen's disease with multiple lateral thoracic meningoceles. Coronal MRI (T-1 weighted in **A,** and T-2 weighted in **B**) shows the CSF-like content of the meningoceles. However, in T-2 weighted image there is a persisting hypointense area (*arrowheads*) to the right, within the largest meningocele. This finding suggests the existence of vegetating associated neurofibroma.

Perineurial Cysts

These were first described by Tarlov in 1938 (52) on the grounds of autoptic observations. The presence of cysts on the posterior sacral roots was considered related to sciatic pain by the same author ten years later. Perineurial cysts typically occur at the junction of the posterior root and the dorsal ganglion, more commonly on the second and third sacral roots, and are frequently multiple. Less common localizations are the coccygeal roots and the dorsal ganglia of thoracic nerves. Very rarely are the cervical root and ganglia involved, although perineurial cysts may be found at any level (Fig. 1.1 A–C). Only sacral cysts may reach a diameter of 1 to 3 cm.

With these cysts pain is nearly always thought to depend on the stretching and compression of the adjacent sensory nerve fibers. The presence of blood in some of these cysts has led to the hypothesis of a traumatic etiology with secondary intracranial hemorrhage. On the other hand, theories of a congenital pathogenesis liken these cysts to arachnoid diverticula of the nerve roots or consider them the result of a splitting of the nerve root sheath, with the formation of a space between the pia-derived endoneurium and the arachnoid-derived perineurium (51). For other authors, however, these cysts arise from a proliferation of arachnoid cells owing to the hydrostatic pressure of the spinal fluid (42,47). The communication with the spinal subarachnoid space is usually poor but nevertheless present (30), in contrast with Tarlov's first experience, which denied any communication.

When small in size perineurial cysts are asymptomatic and are not detectable at radiological examination. Consequently, they are more commonly found at autopsy or accidentally revealed by myelographic or MRI studies. Only the large sacral cysts cause erosion of the anterior and posterior walls of the sacrum, and these are best seen in the lateral projection on plain X-ray examination. However, because of the poor communication with the subarachnoid space, it is recommended to take films at 24 or 48 hours after the administration of intrathecal contrast medium. In the cases where the perineurial cysts do not communicate, a diagnosis may be indirectly reached by the combination of sacral erosion and controlateral displacement of the caudal spinal sac.

References

1. Aarabi B, Pasternack G, Hurko O, et al.: Familiar intra-dural arachnoid cysts. Report of two cases. J Neurosurg 50:826–829, 1979.
2. Agnoli AL, Schonmayr R, Laun A: Intraspinal arachnoid cysts. Acta Neurochir, 61: 291–302, 1982.
3. Amacher AL, Drake CG, McLachlin AD: Anterior sacral meningocele. Surg Gynecol Obstet 126: 986–994, 1968.
4. Ambrosetto C, Alvisi C, Ferraro M: Cisti leptomeningee spinali. Min Neurochir 12:276–279, 1968.
5. Chandler A, Herzeberger EE: Lateral intrathoracic meningocele, case report. Radiology 58:552–555, 1952.
6. Choux M, Yanez A: Arachnoid cysts, in Hoffman HJ, Epstein F (eds): Anomalies of the developing central nervous system. Boston: Blackwell Sci Publ, 1987.
7. Chynn KY: Congenital spinal extradural cyst in two siblings. Am J Roentgenol 101:204–215, 1967.
8. Cilluffo JM, Gomez MR, Reese DF, et al.: Idiopathic ("congenital") spinal arachnoid diverticula; clinical diagnosis and surgical results. Mayo Clin Proc 56:93–101, 1981.
9 Cilluffo JM, Redmond MJ, Ebersold MJ: Idiopathic thoracic intradural and extradural arachnoid diverticula. Report on a case. Acta Neurochir 65: 199–206, 1982.
10. Cloward RB: Congenital spinal extradural cysts. Case report and review of literature. Ann Surg 168:851–864, 1968.
11. Combelles G, Rousseaux M, Dhellemmes P, et al.: Kystes méningés extraduraux rachidiens. Neurochirurgie 29:13–19, 1983.

12. Crellin RQ, Jones ER: Sacral extradural cysts. A rare cause of low backache and sciatica. J Bone Joint Surg [Br] 55:20–31, 1973.

13. Di Sclafani A, Canale DJ: Communicating spinal arachnoid cysts; diagnosis by delayed metrizamide computed tomography. Surg Neurol 23:428–430, 1985.

14. Duncan AW, Hoare RD: Spinal arachnoid cyst in children. Radiology 126(2): 423–439, 1978.

15. Dyck P, Wilson CB: Anterior sacral meningocele. Case report. J Neurosurg 53(4):548–552, 1980.

16. Elsberg DA, Dyke OG, Brewer ED: The symptoms and diagnosis of extradural cysts. Bull Neurol Inst NY 3:395–417, 1934.

17. Erkulvrawart S, El Gammal T, Hawkins J, et al.: Intrathoracic meningoceles and neurofibromatosis. Arch Neurol 36(9):557–9, 1979.

18. Fahrenkrug A, Hojgaard K: Multiple paravertebral lumbar meningocele. Br J Radiol 36:574–577, 1963.

19. Fortuna A, La Torre E, Ciappetta P: Arachnoid diverticula; a unitary approach to spinal cysts communicating with the subarachnoid space. Acta Neurochir 39:259–268, 1977.

20. Gordon AL, Yudell A: Cauda equina lesion associated with rheumatoid spondylitis. Ann Intern Med 78:555–557, 1973.

21. Gortvai P, el-Gindi S: Spinal extradural cyst. Case report. J Neurosurg 26:432–435, 1967.

22. Haberbeck Modesto MA, Servadei F, Greitz T, et al.: CT for anterior sacral and intracorporeal meningoceles. Neuroradiology 21(3):155–158, 1981.

23. Hyndman OR, Gerber WF: Spinal extradural cysts, congenital and acquired. Report of cases. J Neurosurg 3:474–486, 1946.

24. Ivamoto HS, Wallman LJ: Anterior sacral meningocele. Arch Neurol 31(5):345–346, 1974.

25. Kendall BE, Valentine AR, Keis B: Spinal arachnoid cysts; clinical and radiological correlation with prognosis. Neuroradiology 22(5):225–234, 1982.

26. Kim JH, Shucart WA, Haimovici H: Symptomatic arachnoid diverticula. Arch Neurol (Chicago) 31:35–37, 1974.

27. Klenerman L, Merrick MV: Anterior sacral meningocele occurring in a family. J Bone Joint Surg [Br] 55:331–334, 1973.

28. Lake PA, Minckler J, Scanlon RL: Spinal extradural cyst: theories of pathogenesis. J Neurosurg 40:774–778, 1974.

29. Lesbros D, Couilland R, Frerebean P: Kyste arachnoidien intra-dural rachidien. Arch Fr Pediatr 42:309–311, 1985.

30. Lombardi G, Morello G: Congenital cysts of the spinal membranes and roots. Br J Radiol 36:197–205, 1963.

31. Mahboubi S, Schut L: Decrease in size of intrathoracic meningocele following insertion of a ventriculo-venous shunt. Pediatr Radiol 5(3):178–180, 1977.

32. Mapstone TB, White RJ, Takaoka Y: Anterior sacral meningocele. Surg Neurol 16(1):44–47, 1981.

33. Matthwes WB: The neurological complications of ankylosing spondylitis. J Neurol Sci 6:561–573, 1968.

34. Naidich TP, Fernbach SK, McLone DG, et al.: John Caffey Award - Sonography of the caudal spine and back; congenital anomalies in children. AJR 142(6):1229–1242, 1984.

35. Nugent GR, Odum GL, Woodhall B: Spinal extradural cysts. Neurology (Minneap) 9:397–406, 1959.

36. Okamura M, Sumita IC: Cisto aracnoides cervical cirurgico. Seara Med Neurocir 14:143–151, 1985.
37. Palmer JJ: Spinal arachnoid cysts. Report of six cases. J Neurosurg 41: 728–735, 1977.
38. Pan A, Viale Sehrbundt E, Turtas S: Spinal intradural arachnoid cysts. Neurochirurgia 25:19–21, 1982.
39. Perret G, Coreen D, Keller J: Diagnosis and treatment of intradural arachnoid cyst of the thoracic spine. Radiology 79:425–429, 1962.
40. Raimondi AJ, Gutierrez FA, Di Rocco C: Laminotomy and total reconstruction of the posterior spinal arch for spinal cord surgery in childhood. J Neurosurg 75:555–560, 1976.
41. Raja IA, Hankinson J: Congenital spinal arachnoid cyst. J Neurol 33:105–110, 1970.
42. Rexed B: Arachnoidal proliferation with cyst formation in human spinal nerve roots at their entry into the intervertebral foramina. Preliminary report. J Neurosurg 4:414–421, 1947.
43. Robinow M, Johnson GF, Verhagen AD: Distichiasis-lymphedema. A hereditary syndrome of multiple congenital defects. Am J Dis Child 119:343–347, 1970.
44. Roski RA, Rekate HL, Kurezynski TW, Kaufman B: Extradural meningeal cyst. Case report and review of the literature. Childs Brain 11:270–279, 1984.
45. Rubin S, Stratmeier EH: Intrathoracic meningocele. Case report. Radiology 58:552–555, 1952.
46. Schlesinger H: Beiträge zur Klinik der Rückenmarks und Wirbelsäulentumoren. Jena: Fischer, 1898, pp 162–163.
47. Schober R: Cystic formations in the membranous spinal cord covering. Fortschr Roentgenstr 94:116–129, 1961.
48. Smith HP, Davis CH Jr: Anterior sacral meningocele: two case reports and discussion of surgical approach. Neurosurg 7(1):61–67, 1980.
49. Strand RD, Eisenberg HM: Anterior sacral meningocele in association with Marfan's syndrome. Radiology 9: 653–634, 1971.
50. Strully KJ: Meningeal diverticula of sacral nerve roots (perineurial cysts). JAMA 161:1147–1152, 1956.
51. Tarlov IM: Spinal perineurial and meningeal cysts. J Neurol Neurosurg Psychiatr 33:833–843, 1970.
52. Tarlov IM: Perineurial cysts of spinal nerve roots. Arch Neurol Psychiatr 40: 1067–1074, 1938.
53. Teng P, Papatheodorou C: Spinal arachnoid diverticula. Br J Radiol 39:249–254, 1966.
54. Verga P: Di alcune formazioni cistiche della dura madre spinale e della loro interpretazione patogenetica. La Speriment 763:124–147, 1925.
55. Wilkins RH, Odorn GL: Spinal extradural cysts, in Vinken, Bruynn (eds): Handbook of clinical neurology, vol 20. New York: American Elsevier, 1976, pp 137–175.

CHAPTER 2

Syringomyelia and Hydromyelia

Rainer W. Oberbauer

Introduction

The two terms syringomyelia and hydromyelia are frequently used as synonyms or are fused into one expression, syringohydromyelia. Both denote fluid-containing cavities within the spinal cord and are distinguished as either ependyma-lined dilatation of the spinal cord central canal (hydromyelia) or glial-lined spinal cord cavitation with or without communication to the central canal (syringomyelia). They represent morphological findings that brought about a considerable spectrum of attempted etiological explanations (2,42,44,52,73,78,116). Besides many pathophysiological interpretations we may encounter a variety of rare conservative (118) and several operative modalities of treatment (11,15,25,30,48,51,58,77,123), all of which reflect the persistent lack of a conclusive answer regarding treatment of spinal cord cavitations.

In the pediatric population the problem is greater, since symptoms occur mostly in adult life. However, in the vast majority of cases they are due to maldevelopment of the central nervous system (CNS), which occurs in the very first weeks of embryonic existence. Today, it is commonly accepted that hydromyelia and syringomyelia are disorders of circulation of the cerebrospinal fluid (CSF), which occur during the first half of pregnancy and which may be activated by different noxae in later life (12, 25,45,46).

Historical Review

The "prehistory" goes back as far as the 16th century when Estienne, in his "De dissectione partium corporis humani" (1545), gave a description of a cystic dilatation of the spinal cord (37). G.B. Morgagni (1682–1771) initiated exact investigations with his pathological groundwork "De sedibus et causis morborum" in which he portrayed a hydrocephalic case with myelomeningocele and widened central canal of the spinal cord (94).

At that time, some 250 years ago, he drew the remarkable conclusion that hypersecretion of CSF seemed the cause of both the ventricular enlargement and the spinal malformation, thus establishing the first connection between both entities.

The term syringomyelia was coined in 1827 by Oliver d'Angers (100) defining a glial-lined cavity in the spinal cord that may communicate with the central canal or the subarachnoid space (SAS). Bastian (1867) and Strumpell (1880) described progressive neurological disorders years after spinal cord trauma due to development of a syrinx cavity beyond the site of injury (13,121). In 1871 Hallopeau demonstrated, from necropsy findings, unconnected cystic lesions in spinal cords following trauma (60). Leyden (1876) regarded syringomyelia in adults as a remnant of congenital hydromyelia secluding itself from the central canal (82). In 1891 Chiari described two types of hindbrain anomalies still bearing his name (23).

The turn of the century witnessed ideas on operative management and the awareness of different causes of spinal cord cavitation. In 1892 Abbe demonstrated the procedure of syringostomy (1); operative therapy was proposed first by Elsberg (1913) and then, independently, by Borchard (1923) and Puusepp (1923), who proposed laminectomies to perform paramedian incisions of the cysts (19,34,107). In 1936 Frazier reported his experiences with syringostomies (41). The method was extended by Kirgis and Echols (1949) and Love and Olafson (1966), who implanted a tantalum-wire to provide permanent drainage of the cavity (75,86).

In 1874 Simon published his theory of the "Stiftgliome" and suggested that congenital neuroglial hyperplasia formed spinal cysts by degeneration (118). His concepts offered the rationale for radiotherapy for many decades. Joffroy and Achard (1887) gave the first description of adhesive arachnoiditis in syringomyelia (72); Argutinsky (1898) considered the 'terminal ventricle'' in the tip of the conus medullaris as syringomyelia (5). Schlesinger (1902) was first to relate intramedullary cavities to different etiological disorders (115), e.g., trauma, inflammatory leptomeningitis and pachymeningitis, vascular disease, tumors, and malformations of the CNS. Posttraumatic vascular changes with inadequate resorption of degenerate cord tissue were surmised by Minor (1904) as the pathogenetic factors responsible for syrinx formation (93). The possible role of trauma was investigated by Holmes (1915), Collier (1916), and Strong (1919), who found spinal cord cavities as a late consequence of gunshot injuries (24,69,120). Hassin (1920) related the process to primary degeneration with defective glial tissue undergoing abiotrophy (64), and Mackay and Favill (1935) postulated abnormal glial proliferation with subsequent degeneration (37). Vascular insufficiency was reported by Tauber and Langworthy (1935); Netsky (1953) suspected arterial pathology as a causative factor in idiopathic syringomyelia (96,124). The remarkably high incidence of 53% of syringomyelia associated with intraspinal neoplasms was reported by Kernohan (1931). Poser (1956) subsequently found such a correlation in

31% of his patients and concluded that both tumor and syrinx derive from abnormal glial and mesodermal elements in the cord as a result of faulty closure of the dorsal raphé of the neuraxis during embryonic development (74,105). Syringomyelia as part of the syndrome of "status dysraphicus" was often noted by Bremer (1926). Turnbull also (1933) pointed out its frequent association with spina bifida (20,127). The historical enumeration of different theories may be concluded with the thoughts of Grund (1908) and Taylor (1922), who considered CSF pressure and its elevation as decisive factors in the formation of syringomyelia (125).

Embryology

Until the 1950s, etiological explanations for syringomyelia were mainly extrapolations from observations on single cases. Later experimental and clinical investigations succeeded in documenting some of these speculative opinions (22,26,27,31,32,49,50,56,57,73,90,132,134,136), relating the condition of syringomyelia to impaired CSF circulation in combination with dysraphic disorders. McLaurin induced hydrocephalus in dogs by kaolin and found myelomalacia and intramedullary cavities due to adhesive arachnoiditis in the spinal cord (90). As pioneering work we may consider Gardner's hydromyelic theory (46–49), which pointed out that hydrodynamic stresses at the caudad, and less frequently at the cephalad end (where the coverings of the neural tube are most yielding), rupture the neural tube, thus resulting in myelocele. He related cord cavitations to impairment of CSF circulation beginning in the prenatal period.

Normal Development of CSF Spaces

The neural tube closes between the fourth and fifth embryonal week (embryonal length: 4.5 mm) and constitutes the primitive pattern for the cerebral ventricular system and the central canal. The CSF is primarily produced by neuroepithelium and is later secreted by the developing choroid plexus. The ventricular fluid penetrates the permeable rhombic roof to establish and then widen the subarachnoid spaces. As fluid secretion exceeds the absorption capabilities in this stage, the entire neural tube becomes enlarged, and physiological hydrocephalomyelia occurs. The progressive attenuation of the rhombic roof permits increased outflow from the fourth ventricle and reduces the neural tube enlargement even before the apertures of the fourth ventricle become patent. Weed already demonstrated that the sites of the later ventricular apertures represent a primitive ependymal layer with a less differentiated type of cell (130). When the foramina open between the 18th and 20th fetal weeks, the pulsations transmitted to the ventricular fluid by the choroid plexus become diverted from the central canal to the SAS around the neural tube. As a result of this CSF diversion the central canal shrinks and becomes converted into a vestigial structure.

Pathological Development of CSF Spaces

Inadequate permeability of the rhombic roof during the sixth to eighth weeks of embryonal life may not permit sufficient outflow of ventricular fluid from the still obstructed ventricular system, so that the contents of the posterior fossa can be shifted toward the foramen magnum. If the foramen of Magendie remains blocked by an inelastic membrane at the end of the fifth embryonal month, the resultant pressure elevation causes a pressure cone of the soft embryonal hindbrain (Chiari II malformation). If there is the less frequent entity of an elastic membrane occluding the foramen of Magendie, the fourth ventricle becomes cystically enlarged, extending to the cerebellomedullary cistern (Dandy-Walker malformation). In either case the confined pulse waves of CSF remain directed to the central canal and initiate its gradual dilatation (hydromyelia). The pressure waves may damage the ependymal lining of the widened central canal and form a false diverticulum (syringomyelia or syringobulbia) (Fig. 2.1A-C). According to Waldeyer (129), the tendency for dorsal dilation of the syrinx occurs because the posterior columns evolve later than the anterior columns, and the thinner posterior layer of embryonic tissue surrounding the neural tube exerts less resistance. Gardner described a decreasing gradient of CSF pulse pressure from the ventricular system to the lumbar cord (49), which explains the far higher incidence of hydromyelia in the cervical cord right below the herniated portion of the hindbrain. Meningomyeloceles develop if excessive widening of the central canal is confined to few spinal segments.

A subdivision of the central canal may result in diplomyelia and finally lead to diastematomyelia if growth of cartilaginous or bony tissue occurs between the split portions of the cord. Prolonged persistence of the physiological hydromyelia creates secondary widening of the precartilaginous sclerotome leading to a wide spinal canal.

Pathophysiological Concepts

The embryonic malformation of dysraphic states may be the morphological basis for the impairment of CSF circulation gradually leading to symptomatic cord cavitations. The CSF pulse wave is thought to be generated by choroid plexus pulsations. It consists of the steeply rising gradient corresponding to systole and the gradual, diastolic fall (16). It is progressively damped after escaping through the foramen magnum as it passes down the expansible spinal SAS (48). The foramen magnum represents a virtual bottleneck for the CSF as it leaves the rigid cranial cavity. This

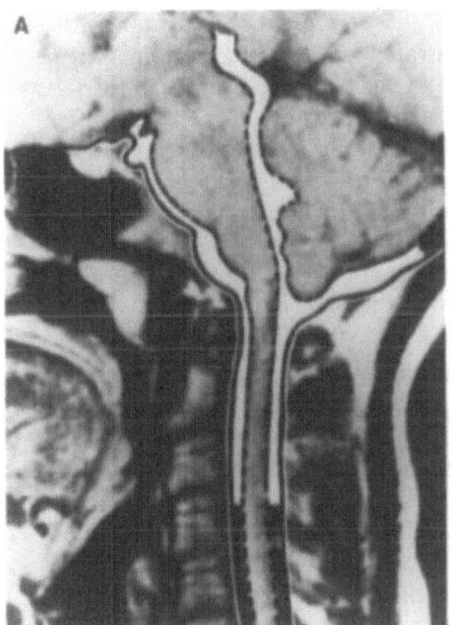
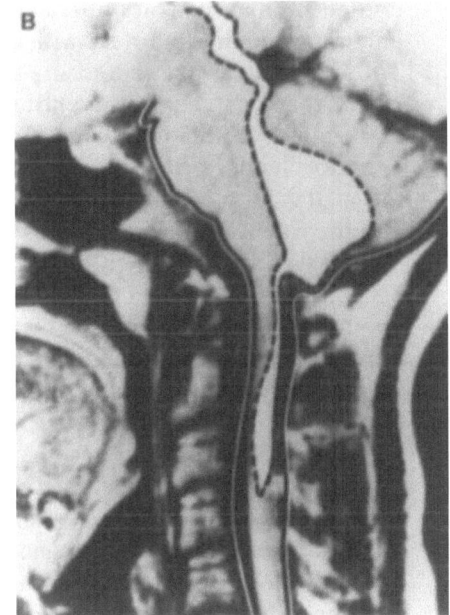
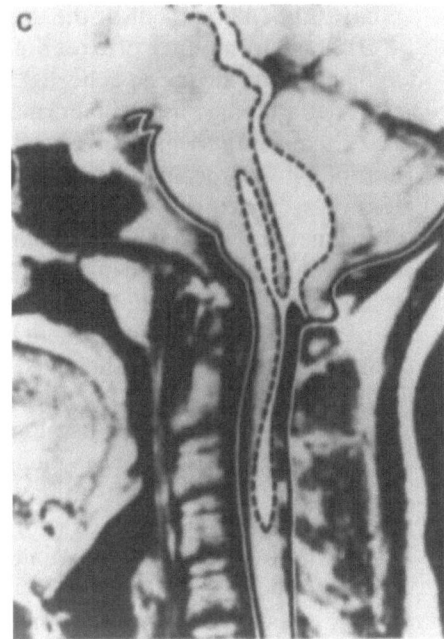

Figure 2.1. A Schematic illustration of normal craniocervical CSF spaces on NMR background. **B** Enlargement of fourth ventricle communicating with cervical syrinx. **C** Syringobulbia plus syringomyelia connected to fourth ventricle.

bottleneck may become obstructed by the downward herniation of the hindbrain and thus interfere with the entrance of CSF into the spinal SAS. The CSF pulse wave then beats to the lower part of the fourth ventricle where the obex marks the entrance to the central canal. If inadequate permeability of the rhombic roof or failing patency of the fourth ventricle apertures hinder CSF diversion from the central canal to the SAS around the neural tube in embryonic life, each CSF pulse wave is transmitted into the patent central canal, thus creating its hydromyelic distention. This is the essence of Gardner's hydromyelic theory, resulting partially from his observation of congenital deformity of the hindbrain in all 74 patients operated on for syringomyelia by posterior fossa exploration, and vertical movement of the impacted hindbrain hernia in response to CSF pulse waves, occluding the foramen of Magendie during the systolic downward excursions. In addition, he observed frequent obstruction of the foramen by a membrane considered to be a persistent remnant of the embryonic rhombic roof. He concluded that syringomyelia represents a dilated central canal being widened by the so-called "water-hammer" effect of each CSF pulse wave propelling a small amount of CSF into the patent central canal. Thus, "the clinical picture of syringomyelia results from progressive, i.e., uncompensated hydromyelia" possibly associated with an unperforated rhombic roof, hydrocephalus, congenital hindbrain herniation, macrocephaly, and enlargement of the spinal canal.

Although a number of experimental, neuroradiological, and operative findings have since been collected to arose qualified doubts and opposition, Gardner's theory of the malformative origin has remained essentially intact. Many authors have observed the same operative finding of hindbrain herniation and occluded foramen of Magendie at the time of posterior fossa surgery but with definitely less consistency (4,62,76,97,110,114,135).

It has been proved from kaolin-induced hydrocephalus with syringomyelia that the central canal was always patent all the way from the obex to the conus (136). Although it may be partially obliterated in the majority of cases later on, the central canal may be open during the developmental stages of this disease in humans. An open communication to the fourth ventricle could be demonstrated radiologically in only 10% (131), and postmortem findings with histological studies supported the rarity of such a patency (12,97,111). Consequently, differentiation has evolved between the communicating and noncommunicating types of syringomyelia (12,30,38,76,103). Compared with the number of studies published on this topic, the evidence of communication is demonstrated by few authors (33,49,65,68,84,85,88,91,101). On the other hand, Gardner's hydromyelic theory presupposes the existence of a patent communication and thus appears rather implausible to explain the pathophysiological relationships in noncommunicating syringomyelia, normal-sized ventricles, or patent fourth ventricle exits.

New hypotheses about possible mechanisms creating hydromyelia and syringomyelia have been published from more recent clinical and experimental investigations (14,17,27,28,56,59,132,133,136). The question whether intracranial arterial pulse waves or intracranial venous pressure changes should be considered as primary distending forces for cyst formation remains controversial. Du Boulay et al. (27) recognized two main pumps generating the pulsatile movements of CSF. The arterial pulse forces blood into the brain and causes expansion of the cerebral hemispheres, particularly the vascular structures. The simultaneously rising intracranial pressure squeezes the third ventricle and forces CSF down the aqueduct and out of the fourth ventricle; in essence, there is a systolic CSF expulsion from the head. He revised Bering's opinion (quoted by Gardner) that the choroid plexus would be the generating force for the CSF pulse waves. The changes in intracranial and spinal venous pressure also act like a pump. On coughing or straining, the spinal venous pressure may well exceed the also increased intracranial venous pressure and contribute to the enlargement of the syrinx once it has developed. From his recordings, Du Boulay accentuates the importance of the basal cistern pulse since its stroke volume is volumetrically ten times greater than the pulsatile waves originated in the third ventricle. The pressure cone of the hindbrain is compared with a ball valve elevating the peak heights of the pressure waves around the brain stem. Such an increased pressure wave may not only force CSF from the fourth ventricle into the central canal, but also create a reflux from the great cistern to the fourth ventricle. This may aggravate the inferior displacement and, possibly, "milk" fluid into the narrow part of the central canal.

The validity of intracranial arterial pulse waves for the distention of cord cavitations has been questioned by Williams (135), who pointed out that noncommunicating syrinxes would also undergo progressive enlargement. In addition, he stated that in a major number of so-called communicating syringomyelia, the narrowed entrance would not allow adequate transmission of pulsatile forces actually to widen the syrinx. He suggested alternatively that the blockage of the SAS at the foramen magnum would be more relevant and that different CSF pressures between head and spine would more likely lead to the distension of the syrinx than would the pulsatile waves propelled to the obex. From his recordings he noted frequently transient differences in venous pressure and termed them "craniospinal pressure dissociation." He explained this phenomenon as a valvelike action at the foramen magnum, caused by pressure differences due to the imposition of energy from the venous system. He also noted that rostral flow of CSF occurs at expiration and that during coughs and strains the lumbar CSF pressure initially exceeds the pressure in the basal cisterns. During coughs or similar pressure elevations, the upward subarachnoid pressure wave compresses the syrinx from below, resulting in a rostral expansion of the cavity. The Chiari malformation permits the rostral flow of CSF into the basal cisterns during venous pressure elevations, and the thus created craniospinal pressure dissociation promotes inferior displacement of the hindbrain and entraps the fluid intracranially. He considers this mechanism as the responsible factor for the formation and enlargement of the syrinx.

A ventriculosyrinx valve effect has also been described from pressure recordings in kaolin-induced syringomyelia by Hall et al. (59). They managed to produce a pressure equilibrium between ventricles, SAS, and syrinx by elevation of the intracranial pressure, but not in the opposite direction so as to increase syrinx pressure artificially. These findings suggested the possibility of syrinx distention by transient elevations of intracranial pressure.

In essence, both intracranial arterial pulse waves and craniospinal dissociations of venous pressure appear to maintain their place in the pathogenesis of spinal cord cavitations. With regard to the variable causes and morphological patterns of this disease we may assume fluctuant connections.

Clinical Aspects

It is a well-known fact that syringomyelia usually becomes symptomatic after the third and forth decades. Reports in children are apparently rare (29,30,43,53,54,70,80,119), except those referring to infants with other dysraphic disorders (35,36,83,89,128). Simultaneous appearance of syringomyelia with spinal cord tumors has also been reported (43,78,105,119). Eggers and Hamer presented a collection from the literature and added two of their own cases for a total of 11 children in about 30 years (30). This obvious rarity of appearance in infancy and childhood seems to reflect the difficulty in recognizing the initial symptoms, which can be confined to paresthetic and sudoral disorders. As one of the very first signs in childhood, kyphoscoliosis has been uniformly described by different authors (30,39,58,68,119). Concomitant to this more or less apparent deformity, clinical symptoms very often start with pain in neck, shoulders, or arms. Dissociated sensory disturbances by impairment of the decussating pathways are considered a characteristic symptom in syringomyelia (Fig. 2.2). Their recognition requires adequate cooperation by the patient and is thus reserved for a certain age. Vasomotor and trophic appearances are naturally easier to detect in childhood. Flaccid motor disturbances reflect the affection of nuclei with respective segmental deficits (Fig. 2.3); the lower limbs are more often involved. Laryngeal paralysis or other cranial nerve disorders originate from syringobulbia. In most cases the course of the disease is slowly progressive (50% to 70%), episodic courses with silent intervals over years followed by possibly rapid deterioration

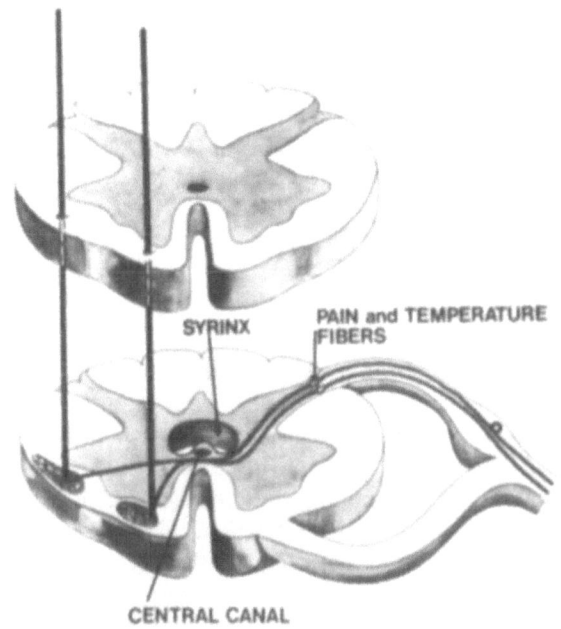

Figure 2.2. Decussating fibers of spinothalamic tract

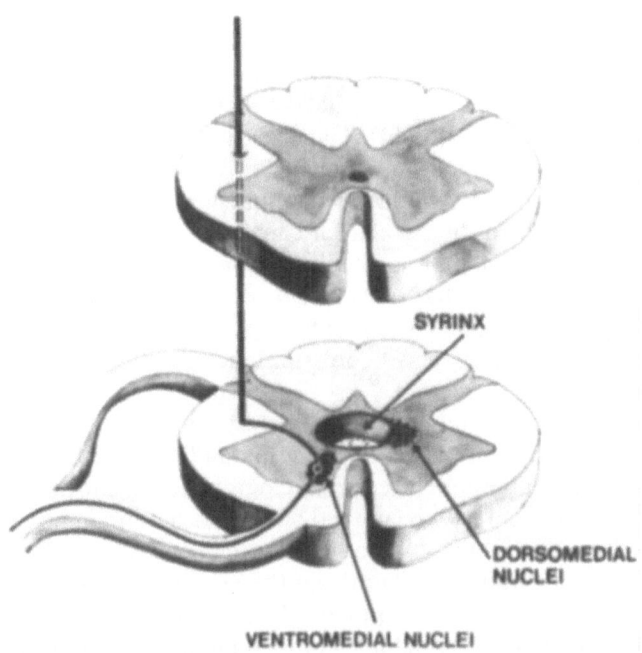

Figure 2.3. Affection of ventromedial and dorsomedial nuclei by the syrinx leading to flaccid paresis in respective segments.

occur in about 30%. Purely rapid progression is seen in less than 10% (30,68,88). Fluid from the cyst is commonly clear and similar in consistancy to CSF. Enclosed cavities may contain fluid with elevated proteintiters, syrinxes associated with neoplasms are filled with plasmalike fluid exuded from the tumor surface.

Neuroradiology

The radiographic investigation is usually started with plain X-ray films of skull and spine, which may show typical abnormalities for this entity. Skull radiography may reveal signs for hydrocephalus, thinning of the calvarium, sellar deformities, short clivus, basilar impression, enlargement of the foramen magnum to accommodate the hindbrain herniation, or stenosis of the foramen magnum. In spinal X-ray films we may find predominantly enlargement of the spinal canal with an increase in the sagittal diameter, (25,63) scoliosis, spina bifida, variations of incomplete fusion of the posterior arch, and block vertebrae (Klippel-Feil deformity) of the cervical spine.

In spite of considerable advances in neuroimaging techniques, e.g., nuclear magnetic resonance, myelography may still be part of the diagnostic management in few instances. Besides the procedures with air or positive contrast medium, the syrinx can be visualized either by direct myelocystography or by filling with contrast via the fourth ventricle. Myelography provides detailed visualization of the intracervical herniation of the tonsils in Chiari malformation and enlarged or collapsed cords according to the head position (down or upright). Harwood-Nash and Fitz demonstrated smooth-walled cysts, which—in combination with the Chiari malformation and the collapsing cord sign due to communicating syrinxes—were considered as enlargement of the central canal, i.e., hydromyelia. They distinguished sausage-string or stacked-coin appearances with scoliosis, but no communication with the fourth ventricle in syringomyelia (63). The latter was related to concentric bands of glial fibers in a circumferential fashion formed by the dissected cord substance creating loculations within the cyst (55).

The collapsing cord sign was described by Conway as evidence for an existing communication between the syrinx and the fourth ventricle (25). As CSF is removed at puncture for myelography, the entrance of air into the ventricular system may be limited due to the hindbrain herniation: the resulting pressure dissociation between cranial and spinal CSF compartments leads to aspiration of fluid from the syrinx, causing it to collapse. In recent years the most widely practiced method has been the combination of myelography with water-soluble contrast medium and subsequent computed tomography (CT) scanning (8,40,108,109,131). By lumbar or lateral cervical puncture the contrast medium is run upward to outline the shape of the cord and possible obstruction of the SAS. Descended tonsils may be identified. Attention must be paid for signs of arachnoiditis around the foramen magnum. About one hour thereafter, cranial CT scans should be performed, with particular attention given to the craniocervical junction. Substantial hydrocephalus is noted in about 30% (3,9,15,45,131). Narrow cuts between the posterior fossa and the level of C-3 are suggested to provide adequate coronal and sagittal reconstructions. At the same time, cuts may be made through the syrinx, which usually reveal a hypodense cavity. Opacification by contrast medium will usually be found after four to six hours; if not, a scan should be repeated the next day. In lateral cervical punctures, the collapsing cord sign and/or a communicating syrinx may be observed by direct, inadvertent puncture of the cyst in larger syrinxes (Fig. 2.4). The collapsing cord sign should not be seen as reliable evidence for communicating syringomyelia (103). The difference in dimensions of collapsed and uncollapsed cord may be appreciated in those patients undergoing this examination because of failure to diagnose the anomaly the first time (Figs. 2.5, 2.6). It is suggested that if contrast medium is seen inside the cyst, or the collapsed cord sign is demonstrated on contrast CT scans, no further investigations should be undertaken (109).

Difficulties may arise from the distinction of purely central cord cavitations and cystic intramedullary tumors (15). We may conclude that the presence of a low-density cyst does not exclude an underlying tumor (Figs. 2.7, 2.8). In their comparative series of cord tumors and syringomyelia, Pullicino and Kendall found enhancement of cord tumors from intravenous

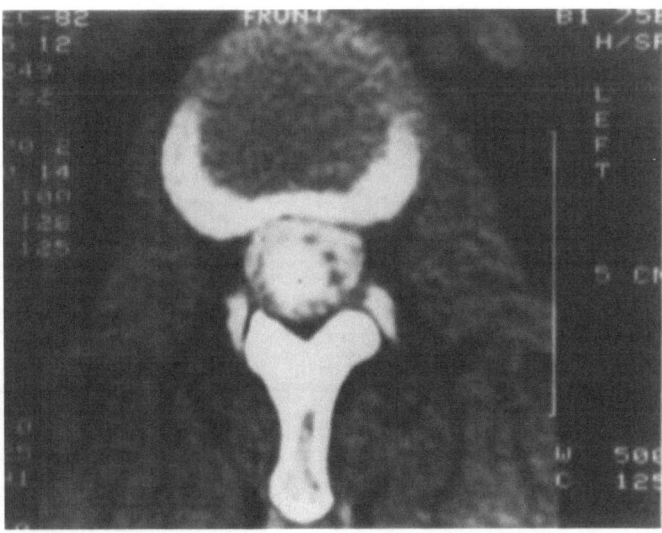

Figure 2.4. Spinal CT scan two hours after myelography. The cyst has extreme concentration of contrast medium.

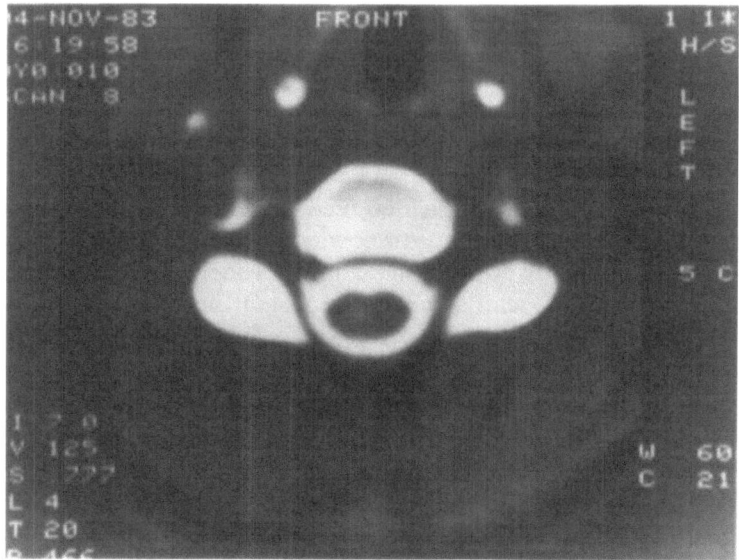

Figure 2.5. CT myelography reveals central cord cavitation with round shape. The cyst is filled by contrast medium.

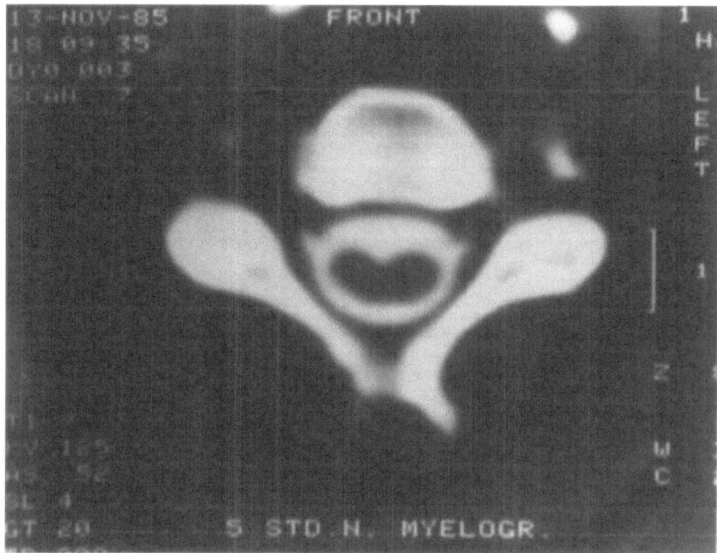

Figure 2.6. Repeated examination in the same patient after 2 years with "collapsed cord."

Figure 2.7. Ascending myelogram with cystic enlargement of the spinal cord.

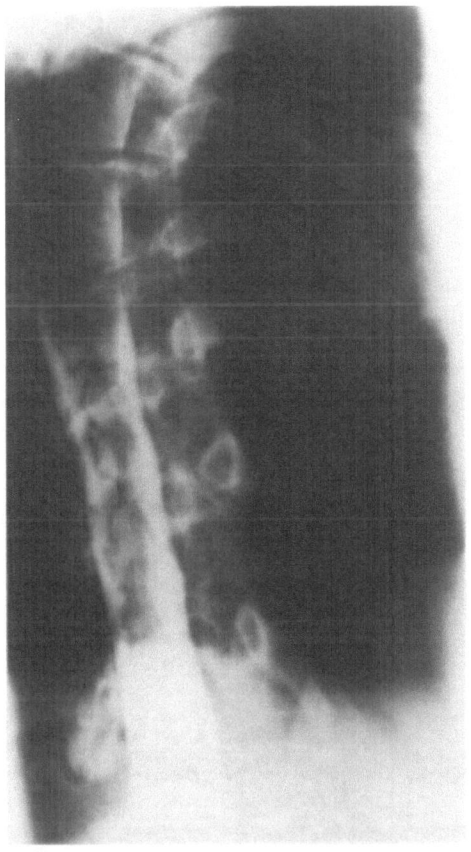

contrast medium injection to be uncommon (106). Contrast medium frequently enters pure cord cavitations but uncommonly opacifies tumor cysts; this feature may be helpful in differential diagnosis, but is not reliable.

The imaging capacities of nuclear magnetic resonance appear to be superior to all current diagnostic methods (Fig. 2.9). It offers distinct appearances of the syrinx and even details like glial fibers forming several loculations within the cyst (Fig. 2.10) (122). The less frequent entity of syringobulbia has been diagnosed clinically but normally missed on traditional radiological investigations. Figure 2.11 shows both a cervical syrinx and a separate, syrinxlike lesion within the medulla oblongata.

Therapy

It is commonly accepted that hydromyelia and syringomyelia are surgical entities that usually require some kind of operative management. There

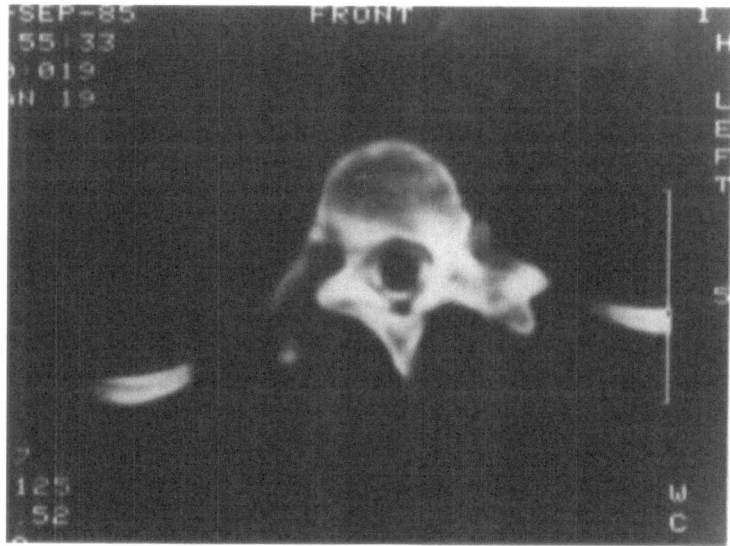

Figure 2.8. Cystic cord dilatation according to previous myelogram. A hemangioblastoma was removed at surgery.

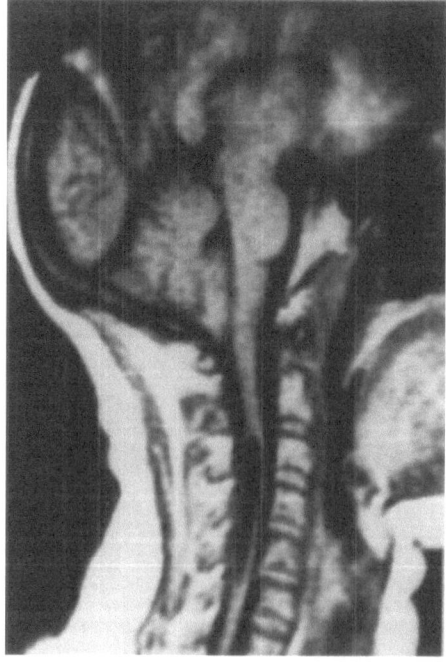

Figure 2.9. NMR with central cord cavitation and Chiari II malformation.

Figure 2.10. Central cord cavitation from NMR; *arrows* point at septations within the cyst.

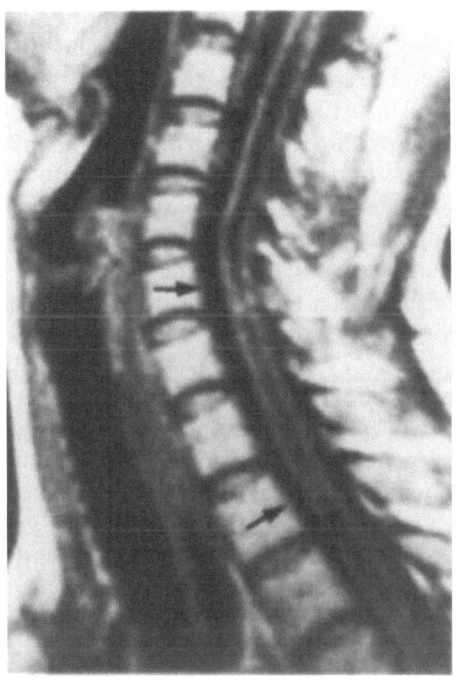

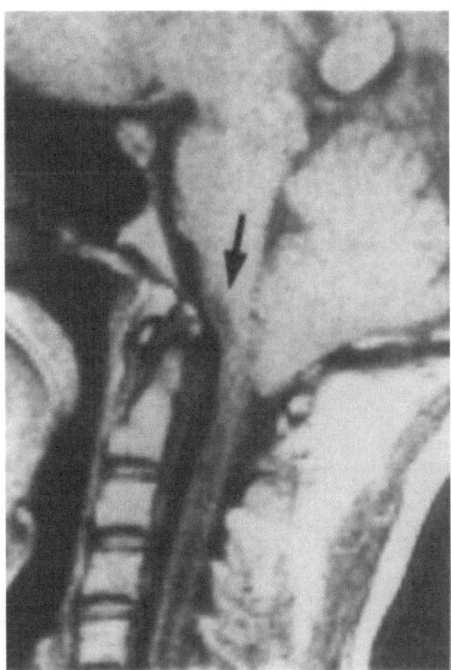

Figure 2.11. Combination of cervical syrinx and syringobulbia (*arrow*).

is no medical treatment. Radiotherapy may be effective in some cystic gliomas, but is generally not considered an alternative therapeutic modality. Percutaneous needling of the syrinx is a possible therapeutic approach (110,113); however, it should be considered rather a diagnostic contribution, as the syrinx most likely will refill after the procedure.

The initial surgical attempts were all directed to the site of the lesion, i.e., the syrinx. The method of syringostomy represented the first serious approach to central cord cavitations, performing laminectomies to incise the syrinx mostly paramedially (15,30,39,110,112,117). Pure fenestration of the syrinx to the SAS provided unsatisfactory results on long-term follow-up. It, consequently, was followed by the insertion of cotton wicks, silk sutures, tantalum wires, or silastic tubes to establish a persistent communication (11,81,86,102,104,123). Myelotomy has since been performed (86,112) and, with some variations, will remain one of the principal approaches. High myelotomy implies the likelihood of increasing the neurological deficit at the site of cord incision, as the cord may be thin-walled and very tenuous. For this purpose, employment of the CO_2-laser is advisable. This promises the most gentle technique for cord incision (Fig. 2.12); furthermore, it may be used to vaporize the glial wall of the syrinx, which may be the site of production of the cystic fluid with higher protein contents (6,7,66,67,99).

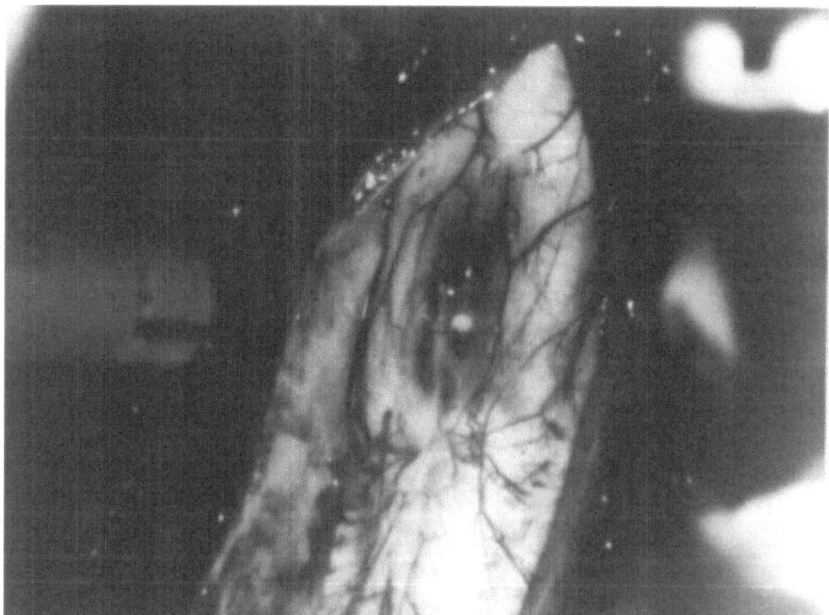

Figure 2.12. Laser handpiece points at cervical cyst. White point marks the pilot laser.

Gardner's hydromyelic theory and his experience with surgical repair of posterior fossa malformations called attention to the hindbrain. He reported his series of 74 patients with the constant operative finding of hindbrain herniation and patent communication between the syrinx and the fourth ventricle. The operative procedure comprises decompression of the herniated hindbrain by posterior fossa craniectomy, fenestration of the frequently occluded foramen of Magendie, and plugging of the patent central canal at the obex. This method has been widely used and accepted by some; however, in other hands operative findings turned out to be less consistent, with higher morbidity and mortality (4,10,44,95,97,135). Krayenbühl suggested the insertion of a muscle plug into the central canal from below by incising the syrinx, a procedure he considered less dangerous (77). The effectiveness of plugging the obex was later questioned, as it was felt by some that decompression of the hindbrain herniation alone by posterior fossa craniectomy and opening the dura would be equally efficient. The value of posterior fossa surgery must also be seen from a historical point of view, as it provided an effective approach to syringomyelia at times when even CSF diversion from the ventricles was still problematic and valve-regulated shunts became just available at that time (98). The introduction of microsurgical techniques has provided more safety in posterior fossa surgery (110), which maintains its place among different operative procedures.

There must have been some incomplete satisfaction with his method since Gardner himself proposed "terminal ventriculostomy" as an alternative surgical procedure. He claimed that there was evidence of tethering in most cases because of a more caudal location of the conus. The procedure consists of excision of the filum terminale together with the tip of the conus. In half of his cases CSF was observed leaking from the cut filum, and either a cavity at the conus or a syrinxlike cavity at the adjoining filum was detected (51,137). Overall experience during some two decades gave rise to other operative modalities, particularly in cases with obvious enlargement of the ventricular system and expected arachnoid adhesions (4,5,28,58,62,76). Complete neuroradiological investigations revealed an average incidence of apparent ventriculomegaly in about 30% (81,131). It was therefore logical to attempt ventriculoatrial or ventriculoperitoneal shunts. Krayenbühl and Benini proposed CSF shunts for communicating syringomyelia as a method with less risk, but not less efficiency (15,76). In cases with evident hydrocephalus and craniospinal pressure dissociation considered unsuitable for posterior fossa surgery, internal ventriculo-subarachnoid procedures may be alternatively employed—e.g., Torkildsen's ventriculo-cisternostomy or catheterization of the aqueduct of Sylvius (79,126).

The development of more sophisticated shunting devices and clear evidence of noncommunicating syrinxes initiated the implantation of tubings into the syrinx, draining into either the spinal SAS (21,123) or into body cavities with lower pressures, e.g., pleura and peritoneum (11,102).

Results

Review of the literature reflects clearly the difficulty with the heterogeneity of this disease and the judgment of the effectiveness of different modes of treatment. Most studies cannot be compared with one another as they employed different initial criteria—including or excluding Chiari malformation, additional etiological factors, and variable and often combined surgical methods. Regarding the variable course of the disease with long stable intervals and sudden accelerating periods, only larger series with adequately long follow-ups appear suitable for comparative judgment. Furthermore, there is insufficient knowledge about the natural history of this entity. In his series, Conway reported six patients refusing surgical treatment, five deteriorating, and one revealing no change in his condition (25). Boman and Iivanainen followed the course of 55 unoperated on patients; gradual progression of the disease occurred in 50%, while the other half remained stable for more than 10 years (18).

Surgical results may be separated according to the primary therapeutic goal, i.e., (a) prevention of filling of the syrinx by posterior fossa surgery and (b) drainage of the fluid collection within the spinal cord or ventricular CSF diversion. The results of the larger series of posterior fossa surgery, including pure decompressive craniectomy, opening of fourth ventricle exits, and plugging of the obex by muscular grafts, are listed in Table 2.1. Results of different draining methods of either ventricular CSF or syrinx contents are summarized in Table 2.2.

Comparison of the two principal surgical modalities reveals no substantiel difference in outcome. Either way, there is improvement in about

Table 2.1. Results of posterior fossa surgery.

Authors	No. of patients	Improved	Unchanged	Worse
Gardner & Angel 1958 (46)	74	70%	15%	15%
McIllroy et al. 1965 (88)	24	33%	38%	29%
Hankinson 1970 (62)	45	82%	0	18%
Barnett et al. 1973 (12)	47	76%	24%	0
Saez et al. 1976 (112)	60	65%	17%	18%
Garcia-Uria et al. 1981 (44)	31	16%	65%	19%
Logue & Edwards 1981 (85)	61	28%	49%	23%
Levy et al. 1983 (81)	85	46%	26%	28%
Total	427	52%	29.3%	18.7%

Numbers in parentheses represent references.

Table 2.2. Results of draining methods.

Authors	No. of patients	Improved	Unchanged	Worse
Pitts & Groff 1964 (104)	28	17	11	0
Love & Olafson 1966 (86)	22	8	9	5
Krayenbühl 1974 (77)	22	13	2	7
Saez et al. 1976 (112)	5	1	2	2
Faulhaber & Loew 1978 (39)	10	2	5	3
Tator et al. 1982 (123)	20	11	4	5
Barbaro et al. 1984 (11)	34	14	9	11
Total	154	69 44.8%	49 31.8%	36 23.4%

Numbers in parentheses represent references.

50%, approximately 30% remain stable, and about 20% deteriorate irrespective of whatever has been attempted surgically. The slight differences between the two methods are to be ignored, as we must consider the different series' variations concerning initial criteria, length of follow-up, and the like.

Synopsis and Comments

The broad spectrum of this disease is best appreciated by considering the great variety of opinions on how to handle this complex entity, including the still existent interpretation of it as a degenerative process for which there is no satisfactory treatment (92). This reflects a rather pessimistic attitude.

Discussing spinal cord cavitations, we must basically separate two different appearances, i.e., first, the form in early infancy associated with spinal dysraphism and, second, the form developing in later life with its variability as to etiology, onset, symptoms, and course:

1. Emery and Lendon (36) demonstrated from necropsy investigations on 100 cases with spinal dysraphism that there is a high incidence of hydromyelia (29%) and syringomyelia (14%) in 43% of cord cavitations cranial to the neural placode. These results are not surprising, as they are clearly supported by experimental investigations in kaolin-induced hydrocephalus, which uniformly presented dilatation of the central canal. As mentioned earlier, the embryonal impairment of CSF circulation inducing the Chiari malformation can be considered a plausible explanation for both hydro-

cephalus and hydromyelia. Gardner suggested that acute hydromyelia alone would lead to meningomyelocele by bursting open the cord. We may, however, additionally assume local, faulty neurulation due to different growth rates of neuroectoderm and mesoderm as a cause of nonclosure or of secondary rupture of the neural tube. It has been demonstrated that extreme cord cavitations may cause considerable damage to the grey matter and, consequently, affect the ascending and descending long nerve tracts (35). This should be expressed clinically by more frequent appearances of neurological lesions located rostrally to the neural placode. However, it can be assumed that cord cavitations in spina bifida represent the communicating type, so that the implantation of ventricular CSF drainage relieves the "hydrocephalus of the cord" at the same time. Thus, hydromyelia, which has often not been diagnosed in the past, remains asymptomatic, as the vast majority of meningomyeloceles (about 90%) require CSF diversions (61). This and the slowly progressive appearance of all other forms of cord cavitations in later life explain the rarity of respective communications in infancy and childhood.

2. Cord syrinxes in later life are encountered on the basis of a number of different causes. Barnett et al (12) distinguished principally communicating and noncommunicating forms and divided this entity into five etiological groups: (a) communicating hydrosyringomyelia resulting from developmental disorders, (b) syringomyelia due to arachnoiditis, (c) posttraumatic syringomyelia, (d) syrinxes associated with spinal cord tumors, and (e) idiopathic syringomyelia confined to the spinal cord.

The first subgroup of developmental malformations may be completed by similar appearances due to adhesive changes in the posterior fossa after perinatal subarachnoid hemorrhage. An extensive investigation of 171 patients with communicating syringomyelia by West and Williams demonstrated that even in this congenital subgroup, only 10% had a radiologically authentic communication between ventricular system and syrinx (131). Although histological examinations (12,97,111) disclosed such a communication with higher frequency, there nevertheless exists a considerable percentage of patients who have no communication. The remaining four subgroups may well be categorized as the noncommunicating type.

The obvious existence of enclosed syrinxes is evidence that Gardner's hydromyelic theory can only be employed for a certain number of syringomyelic cases. As mentioned earlier, other pathophysiological mechanisms must be applied to establish hydromyelia and syringomyelia as explainable entities. Both the pressure cone of the hindbrain acting as a ball-valve and reinforcing the basal cistern pulses toward the syrinx via the fourth ventricle and the craniospinal pressure dissociation of frequently transient differences in venous pressure, may alternate and sometimes compound one another to produce or distend syrinxes in later life.

It is quite clear that in this heterogeneous disease no uniform approach for surgery has been developed. At this point, we may summarize the different possibilities for surgery and present the most commonly expressed objections. Posterior fossa surgery, either decompression, fenestration, or plugging, bears a certain operative risk; the incidence of fatality has been claimed to be as high as 15% (48,62,71,97,135). Some authors reported frequent recurrences, even relapses, after secure blockage of the obex. For cases with arachnoiditis and/or coexisting hydrocephalus, the procedure is not recommended. There is sufficient clinical evidence for myelotomy to go along with some amelioration. It is argued that this observation may be partially due to placebo effects, enforced bedrest after surgery, altered capacitance, or active physiotherapy, but all these possibilities are present for other surgical procedures as well. One of the major disadvantages in high myelotomies—the possibility of increasing the neurological deficit at the site of cord incision—may significantly be reduced by use of more sophisticated instrumentation (6,77,66,99). Although its pathophysiological basis is still unclear, terminal ventriculostomy can be listed among the least risky procedures. But it can hardly be expected to relieve hydrocephalus, and it cannot correct pressure differentials at the foramen magnum or symptoms associated with subarachnoid adhesion in the posterior fossa. There are a number of possible complications from ventricular CSF diversions for ventriculomegaly and communicating syringomyelia. They may require shunt revision but usually imply no substantial risk. Drainages from the syrinx to the SAS are reported to bear a high probability of blockage, and revisions always imply relaminectomies so that their value appears limited (81,123). Some optimism has arisen from syrinx drainage to areas of lower pressure (11,102), although the number of cases and length of follow-up are still insufficient for conclusive judgments.

It is apparent that among the different operative possibilities there is no definitely superior method to handle this variable entity of syringomyelia. Adequate surgical approach can only be evaluated individually according to age, physical condition, morphological and dynamic findings. Opinions about the sequence to be proposed are controversial, and it appears reasonable to set down only basic principles to outline an appropriate surgical attitude:

1. If hydrocephalus is present, it should be treated by CSF diversion.
2. If neuroradiological investigation leaves some uncertainty about diagnosis, myelotomy appears to be the most adequate approach. When pure syringomyelia is proved intraoperatively, a syringo-low-pressure cavity shunt can be performed.
3. Posterior fossa surgery may be favored in all suitable cases with evidence of craniospinal pressure dissociation. If this procedure does not appear feasible, internal drainages, e.g., ventriculo-cisternostomy or canalization of the aquaeduct, may be alternatively employed.

It is a common habit to conclude scientific communications with the sentence that further investigations and experiences are necessary. In the case of this very complex entity, this phrase may legitimately be employed, for there is a particular need for more accurate investigations to aid in the selection of appropriate surgical attitude.

Acknowledgments. The author gratefully acknowledges the radiographic selection by G. Schneider, MD, the secretarial assistance of Mrs Gertraud Machinger, and the preparation of schematic figures by E. Bock.

References

1. Abbe R, Coley W B: Syringomyelia; operation, exploration of cord; withdrawal of fluid. J Nerv Ment Dis 19: 512, 1982.
2. Aboulker J: La syringomyélie et les liquides intra-rachidiens. Neurochirurgie 25(suppl 1): 1–144, 1979.
3. Appleby A, Foster J B, Hankinson J, et al.: The diagnosis and management of the Chiari anomalies in adult life. Brain 91: 131, 1968.
4. Appleby A, Bradley W G, Foster J B, et al.: Syringomyelia due to chronic arachnoiditis at the foramen magnum. J Neurol Sci 8: 451–464, 1969.
5. Argutinsky P: Über die Gestalt und die Entstehungsweise des Ventriculus terminalis und über Filum terminale des Rückenmarks bei Neugeborenen. Arch Mikrosk Anat 52: 502–534, 1898.
6. Ascher P W: The value of recent advances in radiographic and neurosurgical techniques in the removal of spinal canal lesions, in Post Donovan J (ed): Radiographic evaluations of the spine. New York: Masson Publ, 1980, pp 717–721.
7. Ascher P W, Cerullo L: Chapter IX, Laser use in neurosurgery, in: Surgical applications of lasers. Chicago: Year Book Medical Publisher, 1983, pp 163–174.
8. Aubin M L, Vignaud J, Jardin C, et al.: Computed tomography in 75 clinical cases of syringomyelia. AJNR 2: 199–204, 1981.
9. Ballantine H T, Ojemann R G, Drew R G, et al.: Syringomyelia. Prog Neurol Surg 4: 227, 1971.
10. Banerji N K, Millar J H D: Chiari malformation presenting in adult life - its relationship to syringomyelia. Brain 97: 157–168, 1974.
11. Barbaro N M, Wilson Ch B, Gutin Ph H, et al.: Surgical treatment of syringomyelia. Favorable results with syringoperitoneal shunting. J Neurosurg 61: 531–538, 1984.
12. Barnett H J M, Foster J B, Hudgson P: Syringomyelia. London: W B Saunders, 1973.
13. Bastian H C: On a case of concussion - lesion with extensive secondary degeneration of the spinal cord. Proc R Med Chirurg Soc 50: 499, 1867.
14. Becker D P, Wilson J A, Watson G W: The spinal cord central canal: response to experimental hydrocephalus and canal occlusion. J Neurosurg 36: 416–424, 1972.

15. Benini A, Krayenbühl H: Ein neuer Weg zur Behandlung der Hydro- und Syringomyelie. Embryologische Grundlagen und erste Ergebnisse. Schweiz Med Wochenschr 99: 1137, 1969.
16. Bering E A: Choroid plexus and arterial pulsation of cerebrospinal fluid. Arch Neurol Psychiatr 73: 165–172, 1955.
17. Bertrand G: Dynamic factors in the evolution of syringomyelia and syringobulbia. Clin Neurosurg 20: 322–333, 1973.
18. Boman K, Jivanainen M: Prognosis of syringomyelia. Acta Neurol Scand 43: 61–68, 1967.
19. Borchard H: Über die Berechtigung der Operation (Elsberg, Puusepp) bei der Syringomyelie. Arch Klin Chir 170: 94–99, 1932.
20. Bremer F W: Klinische Untersuchungen zur Ätiologie der Syringomyelie, der "status dyraphicus". Dtsch Z Nervenheilkd 95: 1–103, 1926.
21. Cahan L D, Bentson J R: Considerations in the diagnosis and treatment of syringomyelia and the Chiari malformation. J Neurosurg 57: 24–31, 1982.
22. Cameron A H: The Arnold-Chiari malformation and other neuro-anatomical malformations associated with spina bifida. J Pathol Bacteriol 73: 195, 1957.
23. Chiari H: Über Veränderungen des Kleinhirns infolge von Hydrocephalie des Großhirns. Dtsch Med Wochenschr 17: 1172–1175, 1891.
24. Collier J: Gunshot wounds and injuries of the spinal cord. Lancet 1: 711–716, 1916.
25. Conway L W: Hydrodynamic studies in syringomyelia. J Neurosurg 27: 501–514, 1967.
26. Dohrmann G J: Cervical spinal cord in experimental hydrocephalus. J Neurosurg 37: 538–542, 1972.
27. Du Boulay G, O'Connell J, Currie J, et al.: Further investigations on pulsatile movements in the cerebrospinal fluid pathways. Acta Radiol (Diagn) 13: 496–523, 1972.
28. Du Boulay G H, Shah S H, Currie J, et al.: The mechanism of hydromyelia in Chiari type 1 malformations. Br J Radiol 47: 579–587, 1974.
29. Duffy P E, Ziter F A: Infantile syringobulbia. Neurology (Minneap) 14:500, 1964.
30. Eggers Ch, Hamer J: Hydrosyringomyelia in childhood. Clinical aspects, pathogenesis and therapy. Neuropädiatrie 10 (1): 87–99, 1979.
31. Eisenberg H M, McLennan J E, Welch K, et al.: Radioisotope ventriculography in cats with Kaolin-induced hydrocephalus. Radiology 110: 399–402, 1974.
32. Eisenberg H M, McLennan J E, Welch K: Ventricular perfusion in cats with Kaolin-induced hydrocephalus. J Neurosurg 41: 20–28, 1974.
33. Ellertson A B: Semiologic diagnosis of syringomyelia, related to roentgenologic findings. Acta Neurol Scand 45: 385–402, 1969.
34. Elsberg G A: The surgical treatment of intramedullary affections of the spinal cord. Proc 17th Int Cong Med (London) 1913: Section XI.
35. Emery J L, Lendon R G: Clinical implications of cord lesions in neurospinal dysraphism. Dev Med Child Neurol 14: 45, 1972.
36. Emery J L, Lendon R G: The local cord lesion in neurospinal dysraphism (meningomyelocele). J Pathol 110: 83–96, 1973.
37. Estienne C: De dissectione partium corporis humani. Libri Tres. Paris: Simon de Colines, 1945, p 341.

38. Faulhaber K, Kremer G: Neuere Aspekte der Syringomyelie. Pathogenese, Diagnostik, Therapie. Nervenarzt 44:304, 1972.
39. Faulhaber K, Loew K: The surgical treatment of syringomyelia. Long-term results. Acta Neurochir 44: 215–222, 1978.
40. Forbes W St C, Isherwood I: Computed tomography in syringomyelia and the associated Arnold-Chiari Type 1 malformation. Neuroradiology 15: 73–78, 1978.
41. Frazier C H, Rowe S N: The surgical treatment of syringomyelia. Ann Surg 103: 471–477, 1936.
42. Freeman L W, Wright T W: Experimental observations of concussion and contusion of the spinal cord. Ann Surg 137: 433–443, 1953.
43. Gagnon J, Courtois A: Syringomyélie de l'enfant associée à une tumeur intramédullaire. Acta Neurol Belg 60: 37, 1960.
44. Garcià-Uria J, Leunda G, Carrillo R, et al.: Syringomyelia: long-term results after posterior fossa decompression. J Neurosurg 54: 380–383, 1981.
45. Gardner W J, Goodall R J: The surgical treatment of Arnold-Chiari malformation in adults. An explanation of its mechanism and importance of encephalography in diagnosis. J Neurosurg 7: 199–206, 1950.
46. Gardner W J, Angel J: The cause of syringomyelia and its surgical treatment. Cleveland Clin Q 25(1): 4–8, 1958.
47. Gardner W J: Anatomic anomalies common to myelomeningocele of infancy and syringomyelia of adulthood suggest a common origin. Cleveland Clin Q 26: 118–133, 1959.
48. Gardner W J, Angel J: The mechanism of syringomyelia and its surgical correction. Clin Neurosurg 6: 131–140, 1959.
49. Gardner W J: Hydrodynamic mechanisms of syringomyelia: its relationship to myelocele. J Neurol Neurosurg Psychiatry 28: 247–259, 1965.
50. Gardner W J: Myelocele: rupture of the neural tube? Clin Neurosurg 15: 57–79, 1968.
51. Gardner W J, Bell H S, Pooles P N, et al.: Terminal ventriculostomy for syringomyelia. J Neurosurg 46: 609–617, 1977.
52. Gerlach J, Jensen H P: Syringomyelie und Hydromyelie, in: Handbuch der Neurochirurgie, vol 7/1. Berlin-Heidelberg-New York: Springer-Verlag, 1969, pp 335–338.
53. Gerloczy F: Ein Fall von einer im Kindesalter beobachteten Syringomyelie. Kinderärztl Prax 11:88, 1940.
54. Goeters W: Zentrale Gliose (Syringomyelie) bei einem 7-jährigen Jungen. Monatsschr Kinderheilkd 82: 231, 1940.
55. Greenfield J G: Syringomyelia and syringobulbia, in Blackwood W, McMenemy W H, Meyer A, et al. (eds): Greenfield's neuropathology, 2 ed. Baltimore: Williams & Wilkins, 1967, pp 331–335.
56. Hall P V, Muller J, Campbell R L: Experimental hydrosyringomyelia, ischemic myelopathy, and syringomyelia. J Neurosurg 43: 464–470, 1975.
57. Hall P V, Campbell R L, Kalsbeck J: Meningomyelocele and progressive hydromyelia. Progressive paresis in myelodysplasia. J Neurosurg 43: 457–463, 1975.
58. Hall P V, Lindseth R, Campbell R, et al.: Scoliosis and hydrocephalus in myelocele patients. The effects of ventricular shunting. J Neurosurg 50: 174, 1979.

59. Hall P, Turner M, Aichinger St, et al.: Experimental syringomyelia. The relationship between intraventricular and intrasyrinx pressures. J Neurosurg 52: 812–817, 1980.

60. Hallopeau F H: Sur une faite de sclérose diffuse de la substance grise et atrophie musculaire. Gaz Med Paris 25: 183, 1871.

61. Hanieh A, Simpson D A: Cavitation of the spinal cord in association with spina bifida. Z Kinderchir 31 (4): 321–326, 1980.

62. Hankinson I: Syringomyelia and the surgeon, in Williams D (ed): Modern trends in neurology. London: Butterworths, 1970, pp 127–148.

63. Harwood-Nash D C, Fitz C R: Myelography and syringohydromyelia in infancy and childhood. Radiology 113: 661–669, 1974.

64. Hassin G B: A contribution to the histopathology and histogenesis of syringomyelia. Arch Neurol Psychiatr 3: 130–146, 1920.

65. Heinz E R, Schlesinger E B, Potts D G: Radiologic signs of hydromyelia. Radiology 86: 311–318, 1966.

66. Heppner F, Ascher P W: Operation an Hirn und Rückenmark mit dem CO_2-Laser. Acta Chir Austriaca 9: 32–34, 1977.

67. Heppner F, Oberbauer R W, Ascher P W: Direct surgical attack on pontine and rhombencephalic lesions. Acta Neurochir (suppl) 35: 123–125, 1985.

68. Hertel G, Kramer S, Placzek E: Die Syringomyelie. Klinische Verlaufsbeobachtungen bei 323 Patienten. Nervenarzt 44: 1–13, 1973.

69. Holmes G: The Goulstoian lecture on spinal injuries of warfare. Br Med J 2: 769–774, 1915.

70. Huebert H T, MacKinnon W B: Syringomyelia and scoliosis. J Bone Surg 51B: 338, 1969.

71. Jefferson M: Syringomyelia. Practitioner 211: 310–315, 1973.

72. Joffroy A, Achard C: De la myélite cavitaire (observations, reflexions, pathogénie des cavités). Arch Physiol Norm Pathol 10: 435–472, 1887.

73. Kuwamura K, McLone D G, Raimondi A J: The central (spinal) canal in congenital murine hydrocephalus: Morphological and physiological aspects. Childs Brain 4: 216–234, 1978.

74. Kernohan J W, Woltman H W, Adson A W: Intramedullary tumors of the spinal cord. A review of fifty-one cases, with an attempt at histological classification. Arch Neurol Psychiatr 25: 679–701, 1931.

75. Kirgis H D, Echols D H: Syringo-encephalomyelia. Discussion of related syndromes and pathologic processes, with report of a case. J Neurosurg 6: 368–375, 1949.

76. Krayenbühl H, Benini A: A new surgical approach in the treatment of hydromyelia and syringomyelia. The embryological basis and the first results. J R Coll Surg Edinb 16: 147–161, 1971.

77. Krayenbühl H: Evaluation of the different surgical approaches in the treatment of syringomyelia. Clin Neurol Neurosurg 2: 110–128, 1974.

78. Laere J van: Relations de la syringomyélie avec la tumeur médullaire. J Belg Neurol Psychiatr 41–42: 362, 1941/42.

79. Lapras C, Poirier N, Deruty R, et al.: Le cathétérisme de l'aqueduc de Sylvius. Sa place actuelle dans le traitement chirurgical des sténoses de l'aqueduc de Sylvius, des tumeurs de la F.C.P. et de la syringomyélie. Neurochirurgie 21: 101–109, 1975.

80. Lassmann L P, James C C, Foster J B: Hydromyelia. J Neurol Sci 7: 149, 1968.

81. Levy W J, Mason L, Hahn J F: Chiari malformation presenting in adults: a surgical experience in 127 cases. Neurosurgery 12: 377–390, 1983.
82. Leyden E: Über Hydromyelus und Syringomyelie. Arch Pathol Anat 68: 1–26, 1876.
83. Lichtenstein B W: Spinal dysraphism. Arch Neurol Psychiatr (Chicago) 44: 792, 1940.
84. Logue V: Syringomyelia: A radiodiagnostic and radiotherapeutic saga. Clin Radiol 22: 2–16, 1971.
85. Logue V, Edwards M E: Syringomyelia and its surgical treatment. J Neurol Neurosurg Psychiatry 44: 273–284, 1981.
86. Love J G, Olafson R A: Syringomyelia: a look at surgical therapy. J Neurosurg 24: 714–718, 1966.
87. MacKay R P, Favill J: Syringomyelia and intramedullary tumor of the spinal cord. Arch Neurol 33: 1255–1278, 1935.
88. McIllroy R, Richardson J C: Syringomyelia: A clinical review of 75 cases. Can Med Assoc J 93: 731, 1965.
89. McKenzie N G, Emery J L: Deformities of the cervical spinal cord in children with neurospinal dysraphism. Dev Med Child Neurol (suppl) 25: 58, 1971.
90. McLaurin R L, Bailey O T, Schurr P H, et al.: Myelomalacia and multiple cavitations of spinal cord secondary to adhesive arachnoiditis; an experimental study. AMA Arch Pathol 57: 138–146, 1954.
91. McRae D L, Studen J: Roentgenologic findings in syringomyelia and hydromyelia. Am J Roentgenol 98: 695–703, 1966.
92. Merritt H H: A Textbook of neurology, ed 5. Philadelphia: Lea & Febiger, 1973, p 513.
93. Minor L: Traumatische Erkrankungen des Rückenmarkes, in Flateau E, Jackobsen L, Minor L (eds): Handbuch der pathologischen Anatomie des Nervensystems, vol 2. Berlin: Karger, 1904, pp 1008–1058.
94. Morgagni G B: Adversaria Anatomica, book 6, Lugduni Batavorum. Animadvesio XIV, 1740, p 18.
95. Mullau S, Raimondi A J: Respiratory hazards of the surgical treatment of the Arnold-Chiari malformation. J Neurosurg 19: 675–678, 1962.
96. Netsky M G: Syringomyelia. AMA Arch Neurol Psychiatr 70: 741–777, 1953.
97. Newton E J: Syringomyelia as a manifestation of defective fourth ventricular drainage. Ann R Coll Surg Engl 44: 199–214, 1969.
98. Nulsen F E, Spitz E B: Treatment of hydrocephalus by direct heart shunt from ventricle to jugular vein. Surg Forum 2: 399, 1952.
99. Oberbauer R W, Ascher PW, Ingolitsch E, Walter G: Ultrastructural findings in CNS tissue with CO_2-Laser, in: Congr Rep Laser Surgery, vol II. Jerusalem: Academic Press, 1978, pp 81–90.
100. Oliver d'Angers, Ch P: Traite à la moelle épinière et de ses maladies. Paris: Chez Crevot, 1827, p 178.
101. Pendergrass E P, Schaeffer J P, Hodes P J: The head and neck in roentgen diagnosis, 2 ed. Springfield Ill: Charles C Thomas Publisher, 1956.
102. Phillips T W, Kindt G W: Syringoperitoneal shunt for syringomyelia: a preliminary report. Surg Neurol 16: 462–466, 1981.
103. Piscol K, Hamer J: Zur Pathogenese und Therapie der Hydromyelie. Dtsch Med Wochenschr 97: 318, 1972.
104. Pitts F W, Groff R A: Syringomyelia: Current status of surgical therapy. Surgery 56: 806–809, 1964.

105. Poser C M: The relationship between syringomyelia and neoplasms. Springfield Ill: Charles C Thomas Publisher, 1956, pp 98.
106. Pullicino P, Kendall B E: Computed tomography of "cystic" intramedullary lesions. Neuroradiology 23: 117–121, 1982.
107. Puusepp L: Traitement chirurgical de la syringomyelie. Arch Franco Belg Chir 30: 293–309, 1927.
108. Resjö I M, Harwood-Nash D C, Fitz C R, et al.: Computed tomographic metrizamide myelography (CTMM) in spinal dysraphism in infants and children. J Comput Assist Tomogr 2: 549–558, 1978.
109. Resjö M, Harwood-Nash D C, Fitz Ch R, et al.: Computed tomographic metrizamide myelography in syringohydromyelia. Radiology 131: 405–407, 1979.
110. Rhoton A L: Microsurgery of Arnold-Chiari malformation in adults with and without hydromyelia. J Neurosurg 45: 473–483, 1976.
111. Rice-Edwards J M: A pathological study of syringomyelia. J Neurol Neurosurg Psychiatry 40: 198–199, 1977.
112. Saez R J, Onofrio B M, Yanagihara T: Experience with Arnold-Chiari malformation, 1960–1970. J Neurosurg 45: 416–422, 1976.
113. Schlesinger E B, Tenner M S, Michelsen W J: Percutaneous spinal cord puncture in the analysis and treatment of hydromyelia. Ann Meeting Am Assoc Neurol Surg, Houston 1971.
114. Schlesinger E B, Antunes J L, Michelsen W J, et al.: Hydromyelia: clinical presentation and comparison of modalities of treatment. Neurosurgery 9: 356–365, 1981.
115. Schlesinger H: Die Syringomyelie. Wien: Franz Deuticke, 1902.
116. Schliep G: Probleme der Syringomyelie. Fortschr Neurol Psychiatr 47 (II): 557–608, 1979.
117. Shannon N, Symon L, Logue V, et al.: Clinical features, investigation and treatment of post-traumatic syringomyelia. J Neurol Neurosurg Psychiatry 44: 35–42, 1981.
118. Simon T: Beiträge zur Pathologie und pathologischen Anatomie des Zentralnervensystems. Arch Psychiatrie 5: 108–175, 1875.
119. Solheid C: Syringomyélie vraie et gliomatose cavitaire chez l'enfant. Acta Neurol Belg 70: 269, 1970.
120. Strong O S: A case of sacral cord injury and a subsequent unilateral syringomyelia. Neurol Bull 2: 277, 1919.
121. Strumpell A: Beiträge zur Pathologie des Rückenmarks. Arch Psychiatr Nervenkr 10: 676, 1880.
122. Tamaki N, Shirakuni T, Kojima N, et al.: Nuclear magnetic resonance (NMR) imaging in craniocervical anomalies and some surgical considerations. Proc 13th meeting ISPN, 1985.
123. Tator C H, Meguro K, Rowed D W: Favorable results with syringosubarachnoid shunts for treatment of syringomyelia. J Neurosurg 56: 517–523, 1982.
124. Tauber E S, Langworthy O R: A study of syringomyelia and the formation of cavities in the spinal cord. J Nerv Ment Dis 81: 245–264, 1935.
125. Taylor J, Greenfield J G, Martin J P: Two cases of syringomyelia and syringobulbia observed clinically over many years, and examined pathologically. Brain 45: 323–356, 1922.
126. Torkildsen A: Ventriculocisternostomy. A palliative operation in different types of non-communicating hydrocephalus. Oslo: J Grundt Tanum, 1947.

127. Turnbull F A: Syringomyelic complications of spina bifida. Brain 56: 304, 1933.
128. Vuia O, Pascu F: The Dandy-Walker-Syndrome associated with syringomyelia in a newborn infant. Confin Neurol 33: 33, 1971.
129. Waldeyer W: Über die Entwicklung des Zentralkanals im Rückenmark. Arch Pathol Anat 68: 20–26, 1876.
130. Weed L H: Development of cerebro-spinal spaces in pig and man. Washington: Carnegie Inst, 1917.
131. West R J, Williams B: Radiographic studies of the ventricles in syringomyelia. Neuroradiology 20: 5–16, 1980.
132. Williams B: The distending force in the production of communicating syringomyelia. Lancet 2: 41–42, 1970.
133. Williams B: A demonstration analogue for ventricular and intraspinal dynamics (David). J Neurol Sci 23: 445–461, 1974.
134. Williams B: Cerebrospinal fluid pressure-gradients in spina bifida cystica, with special reference to the Arnold-Chiari malformation and aquaeductal stenosis. Dev Med Child Neurol (suppl 35): 138–150, 1975.
135. Williams B: A critical appraisal of posterior fossa surgery for communicating syringomyelia. Brain 101: 223–250, 1978.
136. Williams B: Experimental communicating syringomyelia in dogs after cisternal Kaolin injection. Part 2. Pressure studies. J Neurol Sci 48: 109–122, 1980.
137. Williams B, Faby G: A critical appraisal of "terminal ventriculostomy" for the treatment of syringomyelia. J Neurosurg 58: 188–197, 1983.

CHAPTER 3

Intraspinal Tumors

Concezio Di Rocco, Aldo Iannelli,
and Cesare Colosimo Jr.

Introduction

Despite their relatively low incidence, intraspinal tumors are of considerable clinical interest because of the high percentage of benign and potentially resectable forms, especially in the pediatric population (Table 3.1).

Spinal tumors in children show a slight preference for males (Table 3.2) and for the thoracic segment of the spine (Table 3.3). Many of these tumors are already recognized in the first year of life (Table 3.4).

Anatomical classifications fall into two main groups of spinal canal tumors: extramedullary and intramedullary tumors. The extramedullary tumors can are further subdivided into two subgroups: intradural and extradural. The ratio of intradural to extradural tumors is 3 to 2. Approximately 70% of the intradural tumors in children are extramedullary (5,22,25,50,82,93) (Table 3.5).

The relatively high percentage of benign intraspinal tumors in children may be explained by the frequency with which tumors associated with dysraphia or split notochord lesions become symptomatic in the first years of life (43,49). The tumors that occur in the pediatric age group and are not maldevelopmental in origin are those primarily located within the spinal cord. Most extramedullary tumors occurring in children are those developing in the epidural space, those resulting from seeding of neoplastic cells through the cerebrospinal fluid (CSF), and those originating from blood vessels, meninges, nerve roots, and vertebrae (8).

It is worth noting, however, that several types of tumors, such as teratomas, dermoids, and epidermoids, may be extramedullary and intramedullary at the same time. In particular, the ependymoma is commonly intramedullary when it occurs at the conus medullaris, although it is almost entirely extramedullary within the dural sac at the level of the cauda equina.

Table 3.1. Spinal tumor types.

Study	Gliomas (%)	Sarcomas (%)	Neuroblastomas, ganglioneuromas (%)	Neurinomas, neurofibromas (%)	Meningiomas (%)	Dermoids (%)	Lipomas (%)	Others (%)
Haft et al. 1959 (49)	30.0	13.4	30.0	6.7	3.3	13.3	—	3.3
Rand et al. 1960 (93)	41.6	20.8	12.5	10.4	4.2	4.2	2.1	4.2
Arseni et al. 1967 (4)	31.4	25.7	2.9	20.0	5.7	14.3	—	—
Banna et al. 1971 (8)	39.1	17.4	34.8	8.7	—	—	—	—
Grote et al. 1975 (47)	25.3	19.3	2.4	13.2	2.4	16.9	13.2	7.3
Kordas et al. 1977 (59)	21.2	25.8	4.5	9.1	—	18.2	3.0	18.2
De Sousa et al. 1979 (22)	22.2	13.6	7.4	11.1	3.7	9.9	9.9	22.2
Di Lorenzo et al. 1982 (25)	19.6	16.1	28.6	7.1	—	7.1	1.8	19.7
Hendrick, 1982 (55)	22.5	3.8	11.3	5.0	—	13.8	1.2	42.4
Hahn et al. 1984 (50)	27.8	27.8	—	—	—	5.6	9.3	29.5

Table 3.2. Sex distribution.

Study	Males (%)	Females (%)
Hamby 1944 (51)	57.9	42.4
Haft et al. 1959 (49)	56.7	43.3
Rand et al. 1960 (93)	61.9	38.1
Arseni et al. 1967 (4)	50.0	50.0
Grote et al. 1975 (47)	47.0	53.0
De Sousa et al. 1979 (22)	59.3	40.7
Di Lorenzo et al. 1982 (25)	48.2	51.8
Hendrick 1982 (55)	63.7	36.3
Hahn et al. 1984 (50)	51.8	48.2

Table 3.3. Spinal segment.

Study	C (%)	C–T (%)	T (%)	T–L (%)	L (%)	L–S (%)	S (%)	Multiple levels (%)
Hamby 1944 (51)	21.0	5.3	36.9	8.8	7.9	9.6	1.7	8.8
Rand et al. 1960 (93)	10.2	8.2	34.7	12.2	6.1	20.4	4.1	4.1
Arseni et al. 1967 (4)	—	8.3	58.3	33.4	—	—	—	—
Grote et al. 1975 (47)	11.5	5.1	47.4	—	16.8	11.5	7.7	—
Kordas et al. 1977 (59)	21.2	5.0	35.0	11.3	5.0	18.8	—	3.7
De Sousa et al. 1979 (22)	29.6	—	27.2	—	32.1	—	11.1	—
Di Lorenzo et al. 1982 (25)	23.1	5.4	30.4	16.1	14.3	7.1	1.8	1.8
Hendrick 1982 (55)	13.7	2.5	25.0	17.6	31.2	—	3.7	6.3
Hahn et al. 1984 (50)	15.2	—	45.8	—	30.5	—	8.5	—

Table 3.4. Age distribution (yr).

Study	0–1 (%)	1–2 (%)	2–3 (%)	3–4 (%)	4–5 (%)	5–6 (%)	6–7 (%)	7–8 (%)	8–9 (%)	9–10 (%)	10–11 (%)	11–12 (%)	12–13 (%)	13–14 (%)	14–15 (%)	15–16 (%)
Hamby 1944 (51)	5.5	1.5	8.5	3.4	5.5	3.4	8.0	6.0	7.0	4.0	6.0	7.5	6.5	14.4	12.8	—
Haft et al. 1959 (49)	20.0	—	10.0	13.2	—	6.7	—	—	6.7	10.0	6.7	10.0	6.7	—	10.0	—
Rand et al. 1960 (93)	18.3	8.2	4.1	6.1	4.1	4.1	4.1	8.2	6.1	2.0	12.2	8.2	8.2	4.1	2.0	—
Grote et al. 1975 (47)	15.1	9.6	9.6	1.4	4.1	4.1	2.7	6.8	2.7	2.7	4.1	1.4	8.2	5.5	8.3	13.7
Kordas et al. 1977 (59)	2.5	13.7	11.2	8.8	5.0	8.8	8.8	8.8	1.2	1.2	7.5	8.8	6.2	7.5	—	—
Di Lorenzo et al. 1982 (25)	16.0	10.7	12.5	5.4	1.8	—	7.1	3.6	7.1	3.6	3.6	5.4	12.5	10.7	—	—
Hendrick 1982 (55)	2.5	12.7	10.2	2.5	10.2	3.8	6.3	7.6	7.6	7.6	3.8	7.6	2.5	6.3	6.3	2.5

Table 3.5. Site localization.

Authors	Total number	Intramedullary	Intradural	Extradural	Extraintradural
Hamby 1944 (51)	185	27.3	33.6	38.2	0.9
Haft et al. 1959 (49)	30	33.3	16.7	50.0	—
Rand et al. 1960 (93)	48	41.6	16.7	39.6	2.1
Arseni et al. 1967 (4)	35	38.1	33.3	28.6	—
Banna et al. 1971 (8)	23	39.1	8.7	52.2	—
Grote et al. 1975 (47)	83	25.3	15.7	59.0	—
Kordas et al. 1977 (59)	66	35.0	25.0	40.0	—
De Sousa et al. 1979 (22)	70	28.4	37.0	34.6	—
Di Lorenzo et al. 1982 (25)	56	19.6	17.9	62.5	—
Hahn et al. 1984 (50)	54	22.3	37.0	40.7	—
McLaurin 1984 (71)	—	33	67%		

Clinical Symptoms and Signs

The combination of (a) symptoms of local neural damage and disturbances related to the involvement of the longitudinally running ascending and descending tracts and (b) interruption of the functions below the level of the lesion characterizes the clinical manifestations of intraspinal tumors in children, as it does in adults.

The extramedullary location of a mass expanding within the spinal canal on one side of the spinal cord is clinically revealed by unilateral neurological deficits, with a relatively frequent occurrence of Brown-Séquard's syndrome.

Conversely, the intramedullary location is typically manifested by a dissociated sensory loss due to the interruption of the crossing pain fibers and when involving the spinothalamic tracts, by the relative sparing of the more externally placed lumbosacral fibers, which conduct pain and temperature. This theoretical distinction is unfortunately not always apparent in clinical practice. In fact, in most patients the symptomatology is more obviously influenced by the cervicothoracic or lumbosacral level of the lesion rather than by its spatial relationship with the neural spinal structures in the axial plane.

Furthermore, in almost all cases of intraspinal tumors, the recognition of an extramedullary or intramedullary location of a tumor, on clinical grounds alone, is made difficult by the significant delay in diagnosis that is usually experienced. Indeed, in most patients the clinical manifestations may precede the actual discovery of the lesion by several months or even years (5,50,106).

Pain is the predominant isolated complaint in both intramedullary and extramedullary localizations. The symptom is described as either vertebral, radicular, or medullary (remote, funicular, or referred pain). Its intensity usually increases during sleep, with strain, or after Valsalva's maneuver. Pain is also the most frequent and the most common initial complaint (8,49,50,82) (Table 3.6), although it is often neglected or misinterpreted in young subjects. Pain, in fact, may be interpreted as due to torticollis when occurring in the cervical region and to "growth" when located at the lumbar level (5).

Radicular pain may be relatively frequent, especially in the lower limbs. This symptom is often regarded as suggestive of an extramedullary lesion, although it occurs also in intramedullary lesions. The intensity of radicular pain may be great and is usually described as similar to that of cramps or electrical discharges (49).

In some children with low thoracic spinal tumors, the occurrence of radicular pain often leads to the misdiagnosis of an abdominal lesion, especially when the T-11 root is involved. Psychological problems may be propounded in interpreting the discrete radicular pain that characterizes tumors of the cauda equina, which selectively impair one single dorsal

Table 3.6. Clinical signs.

	De Sousa et al. 1979 (22) (%)	Hendrick 1982 (55) (%)	Hahn et al. 1984 (50) (%)
Pain	50.6	36.3	78.0
Motor weakness	55.5	65.0	76.0
Reflex changes	56.8	75.0	74.0
Sensory disturbance	40.7	55.0	50.0
Spasticity	12.4	—	37.0
Sphincter involvement	30.8	33.7	30.8
Spine tenderness	9.8	46.3	24.0
LSLR	6.0	26.2	15.0
Gait disturbance	65.5	—	11.0
Scoliosis	11.0	32.5	9.0
Muscle atrophy	9.8	—	7.0
Café-au-lait spot	7.4	—	2.0
Symptoms of SAH	—	3.7	—
Papilledema	—	2.5	—

LSLR = limitation straight leg raising; SAH = subarachnoid hemorrhage.

root. The pain assumes a clear diagnostic value only when associated with obvious *deformities of the spinal column*. These deformities include scoliosis, with either a simple or double curvature, kyphosis, and stiffness of the spine (5). The last abnormality, although occurring relatively late in the course of the disease, may be so severe, particularly in infants, as to induce hyperlordosis, opisthotonos, or even torsion of the spine simulating a dystonic condition (Fig. 3.1).

Motor weakness, especially of the lower but also of the upper limbs, frequently constitutes the presenting sign of a spinal tumor in the newborn (65) and is second only to pain as the most frequent presenting symptom in infancy and childhood (107). Nevertheless, motor deficits may long remain absent or discrete in older children. When clinically apparent, they are frequently confined to the lower limbs in the form of gait disturbances and deformities of the feet (Fig. 3.2) often calling for the attention of the orthopedic surgeon. Bilateral weakness and growth deformities may be more commonly localized to only one side and accompanied by obvious muscular atrophy in some patients.

Paresthesia and *sphincter disturbances* are rare in children. Disturbances in micturition, which in toilet-trained children may suggest a caudal spinal tumor, are difficult to evaluate in infants. Enuresis, deformities of the lower limbs, and gait disturbances acquire definite diagnostic value when associated with abnormalities of the lumbar region, such as the evidence of a dermal sinus and areas of hairy or pigmented cutaneous lesions.

Conversely, other symptoms, which have been reported in children with spinal tumors, have an aspecific and potentially confusing significance for the diagnosis. They include meningeal signs, headache, abdominal dis-

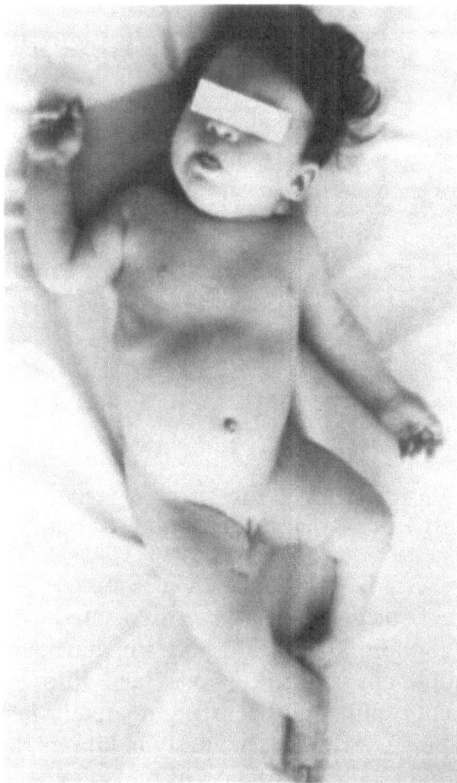

Figure 3.1. Severe stiffness of the spine simulating a dystonic condition.

comfort, and bowel paralysis, as well as fever and deterioration of the condition in general (5,46,71) (Table 3.7).

The high incidence of an associated obstructive or communicating hydrocephalus, which in children may be as much as 14% (71), is of particular interest. Hydrocephalus is found in cases of either intramedullary, intradural, extramedullary, or extradural tumors and is thought to depend on different factors, such as arachnoiditis (4,68), a tentorial or cisternal

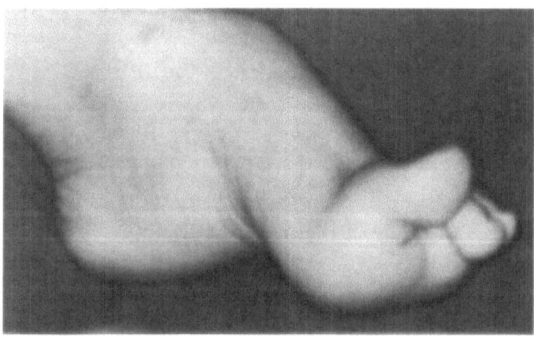

Figure 3.2. Deformity of the feet resulting from long-standing spinal tumor.

Table 3.7. Unusual clinical manifestations of spinal tumors.

1. Acute onset of transectional dysfunction and flaccid paralysis.
2. Acute onset with signs of subarachnoid hemorrhage.
3. Exceptionally rapid (hours) or slow (years) progression of clinical deterioration.
4. Cranial nerve involvement.
5. Papilledema and/or hydrocephalus.
6. Nystagmus.

After Stern (107), with modifications.

block in CSF circulation (77), increased protein content (52), and subarachnoid hemorrhages.

Course of Symptoms

The evolution of the clinical manifestations of spinal tumors is progressive, although characterized in some cases by an intermittent course. Nevertheless, an unusually rapid deterioration of the clinical condition, in a matter of hours, can be observed even in children with benign lesions.

Before the introduction of computed tomography (CT) and magnetic resonance imaging (MRI) techniques, the progression of symptoms was an important factor in the formulation of a diagnosis. Four main subsequent stages could be distinguished: (a) early neuralgia characterized by pain, (b) a Brown-Séquard pattern of deficits, (c) an incomplete and then (d) complete transectional dysfunction (24). However, a diagnosis based on the progression of clinical deterioration was unsatisfactory and often too late, as half the patients usually progressed to total sensorimotor paralysis before surgical treatment was carried out (107). Pitfalls in diagnosis were common, especially with peripheral neuritis or demyelinating diseases. Furthermore, additional difficulties had to be faced when the clinical presentation of the tumor or its evolution assumed unusual clinical features (Table 3.7).

Basic Neuroradiology of Spinal Mass Lesions

During the past decade neuroradiology has moved from conventional studies to the modern and exciting neuroimaging, with the introduction and wide diffusion of CT, ultrasonography (US), and, more recently, MRI. In the field of spinal diagnoses the new imaging modalities represent an invaluable advantage, and today spinal mass lesions may be rapidly diagnosed by means of relatively noninvasive methods. Although a histological definition is not yet possible in many cases without surgical exploration, most patients are operated on with a good radiological suggestion of the nature of the tumor; continuous progress in tissue characterization (by CT, US, and above all, MRI) leads us to expect even superior results in the near future.

The complete spectrum of neuroradiological procedures for the diagnosis of spinal "tumors" includes standard X-ray studies (with tomography), radionuclide studies (RNS), US, myelography, CT, MRI, and even angiography. A redefinition of the capabilities of each method can now be useful in planning an up-to-date rational protocol.

A standard X-ray study of the spine is still the first radiological step in the evaluation of a child with a suspected spinal mass lesion. The whole spine must be examined in sagittal and coronal projections. The following basic pathological findings may be found:

1. Acquired structural bony changes, usually osteolytic and rarely sclerotic. Primary and secondary tumors of the bony vertebrae are the most frequent causes of the destructive vertebral lesions (Fig. 3.3).

2. Local or generalized enlargement of the spinal canal. This is the most typical finding. An obvious thinning of the medial surfaces of the pedicles, with increased interpedunculate distance, as well as severe scalloping of the posterior vertebral bodies (Fig. 3.4A), strongly suggests an intraspinal expanding lesion; however, in neonates and younger children a minimal

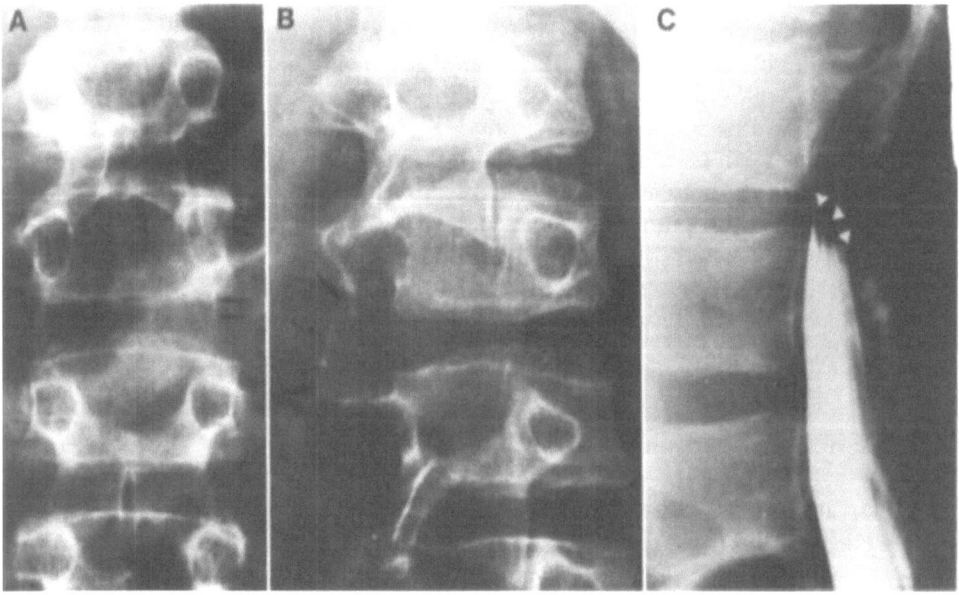

Figure 3.3. Chondrosarcoma involving laminae, spinous process and inferior articular pillars of L-2 with obvious signs of mass lesion. **A,B** Standard AP and oblique views reveal the bony destructive changes and the calcified borders of the tumor (*arrows*). **C** Myelography shows a complete extradural block. The dural sac is compressed and displaced anteriorly (*arrowheads*).

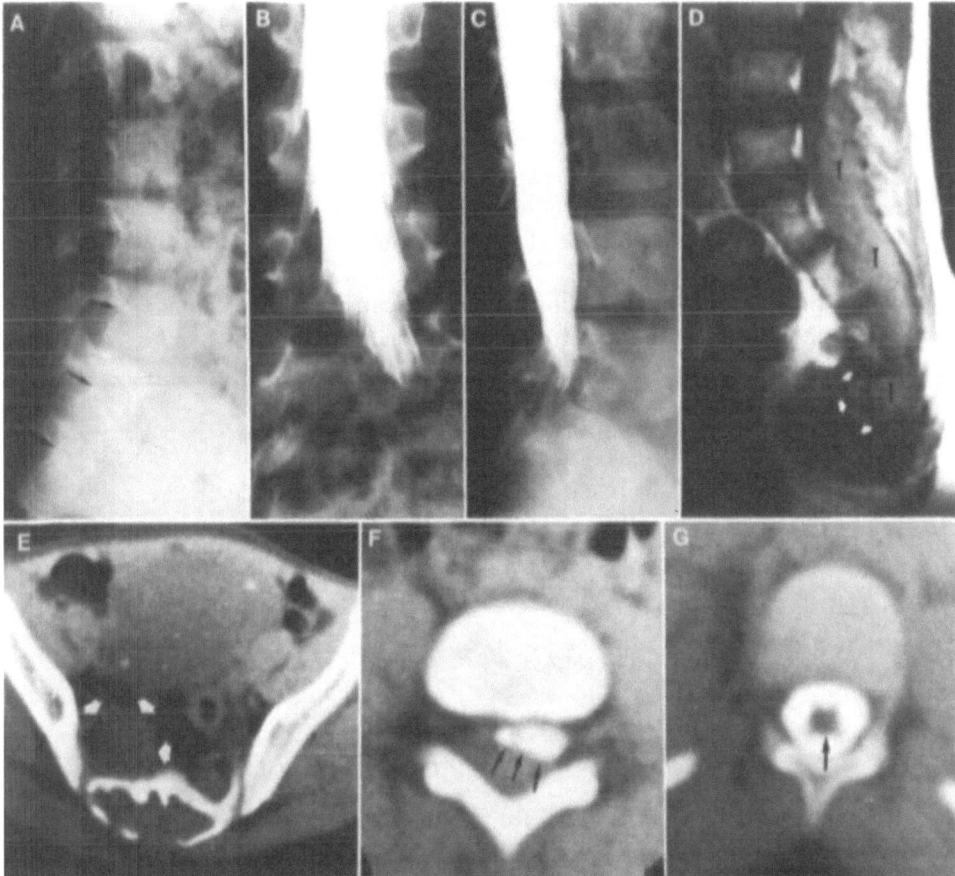

Figure 3.4. Giant neurinoma of the cauda equina in a 10-year-old boy with a long history of paraparesis and gait disturbances. **A** Standard lateral view of the lumbosacral spine reveals severe scalloping of the lumbosacral vertebral bodies (*arrows*). **B,C** Myelography demonstrates a large extradural mass displacing anteriorly and toward left the dural sac. **D** Sagittal T1-weighted MRI shows the tumor (T), hyperintense in comparison with the CSF, extending from L-4 to the lower sacral vertebra and protruding anteriorly within the pelvis (*arrows*). **E** CT scan confirms the tumor eroding the sacral bone and occupying the sacral canal and foramina as well as bulging in the right pelvis (*arrows*). **F** Myelo-CT depicts the relationships between the tumor and the dural sac (*arrows* at L-5. **G** The conus medullaris is completely normal (*arrow*).

degree of expansion is not easy to detect because of the "physiologic enlargement" of the spinal canal in comparison with older children and teenagers. Therefore, it must be kept in mind that the spinal canal/vertebral body ratio progressively decreases from birth to the adult age (53,54). Furthermore, other conditions (i.e., neurofibromatosis, mucopolysaccharidosis) may cause spinal canal enlargement without intraspinal expansile lesions. Conversely, enlargement of one or more intervertebral foramina represents a reliable sign of a foraminal mass lesion (Fig. 3.5).

3. Paraspinal abnormalities. Soft tissue or denser masses are easily detected on plain films of the thoracic area because of the air lung contrast and anatomical landmarks of pleural mediastinal lines (Fig. 3.6). X-ray

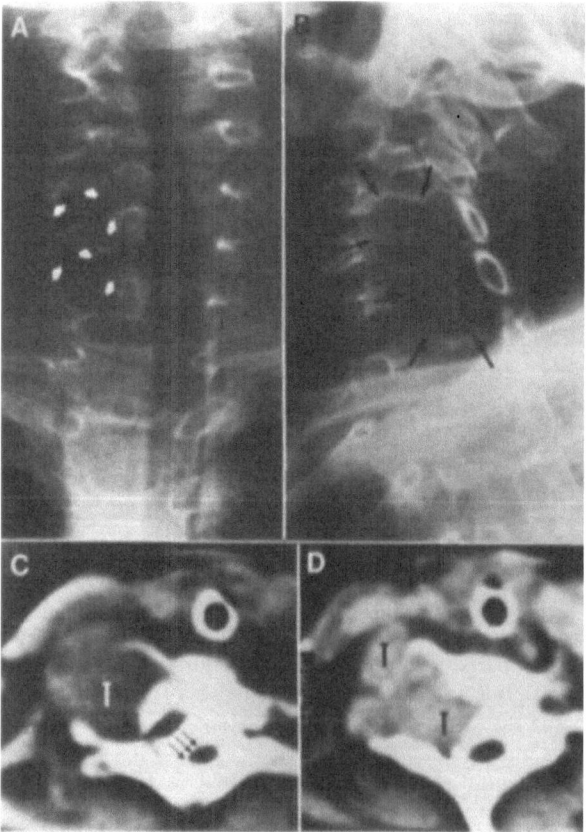

Figure 3.5. Hourglass neurinoma extending into the brachial plexus in a child without any neurologic symptom. **A,B** Anteroposterior and oblique films of the cervical spine demonstrate obvious enlargement of the C-5 to C-6 and C-6 to C-7 neuroforamina (*arrows*). **C** Myelo-CT depicts the tumor mass (T) with intraspinal extradural involvement and mild cord compression (*arrows*). **D** After further intravenous administration of contrast medium, the tumor (T) is clearly enhanced, and its extension within the enlarged neuroforamen is better outlined.

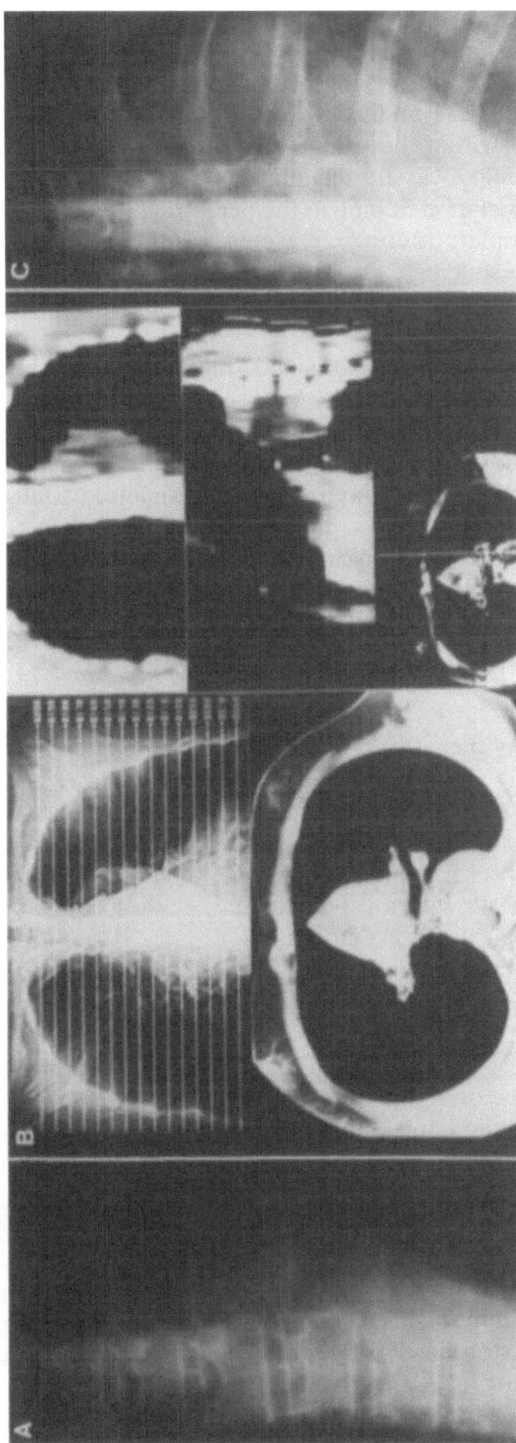

Figure 3.6. Thoracic paraspinal ganglioneuroma without intraspinal invasion. **A** Plain film shows scoliosis as well as left paraspinal mass. **B** CT scan well defines the shape and relationships of the tumor. **C** Myelography confirms the absence of intraspinal involvement.

recognition of a paraspinal mass in the lower thoracic, lumbar, and pelvic areas is possible but more difficult; a cervical mass is easier to detect by palpation than by x-ray films.

4. Calcifications. These findings are very significant, and even small deposits of calcium within the spinal canal or in the paraspinal regions must be checked using a careful technique.

5. Dysraphia. A common finding in the pediatric population, dysraphia ranges from the simple posterior rachischisis to the most total complex and sometimes grotesque pictures. A dysraphic abnormality is frequently encountered as the unique X-ray finding for maldevelopmental mass lesions (Fig. 3.7).

6. Postural abnormalities. These include modifications in both sagittal and coronal alignment of the spine. Loss of the normal lordosis in the lumbar or cervical spine has the same significance as an acquired unexplained scoliosis, and both conditions may be the most impressive x-ray finding of an underlying spinal tumor (especially an intramedullary lesion) (Figs. 3.6, 3.8A).

Obviously many other pathological conditions result in pain and postural changes, and only a skillful clinical evaluation guides the specialist to the recognition of the spinal or extraspinal source of symptoms.

Radionuclide Studies

Bone scintigraphy by means of technetium 99 is employed in all cases in which structural bony changes are evident on standard x-ray films in order to exclude multiple lesions (53). Multiple localizations are not unusual in children with, for example, histiocytosis X, leukemia, metastatic neuroblastomas, or Ewing's sarcoma. In such cases RNS have little specificity but high sensitivity, allowing a diagnosis of multiple localizations before a clinical or radiological manifestation.

Ultrasonography

The introduction of specialized "small parts" transducers (high-frequency 7.5 mHz linear or sectorial) makes spinal US studies in children possible (57, 86). Basically, sonograms of the pediatric spine are useful only up to 6 months of age because the lack of fusion of the posterior elements results in an acoustic window through which to explore the spinal canal and its content. Later on spinal US is possible only when there is a wide rachischisis or laminectomy "opening" an acoustic window.

In the newborn, US, using a sagittal plane, clearly depicts the hypoechoic spinal cord within the spinal canal, and high-resolution transducers facilitate the demonstration of the central echogenic canal; in the lumbar tract the filum terminalis and the roots of the cauda equina may also be seen. Because of the low frequency of true spinal cord tumors in the first

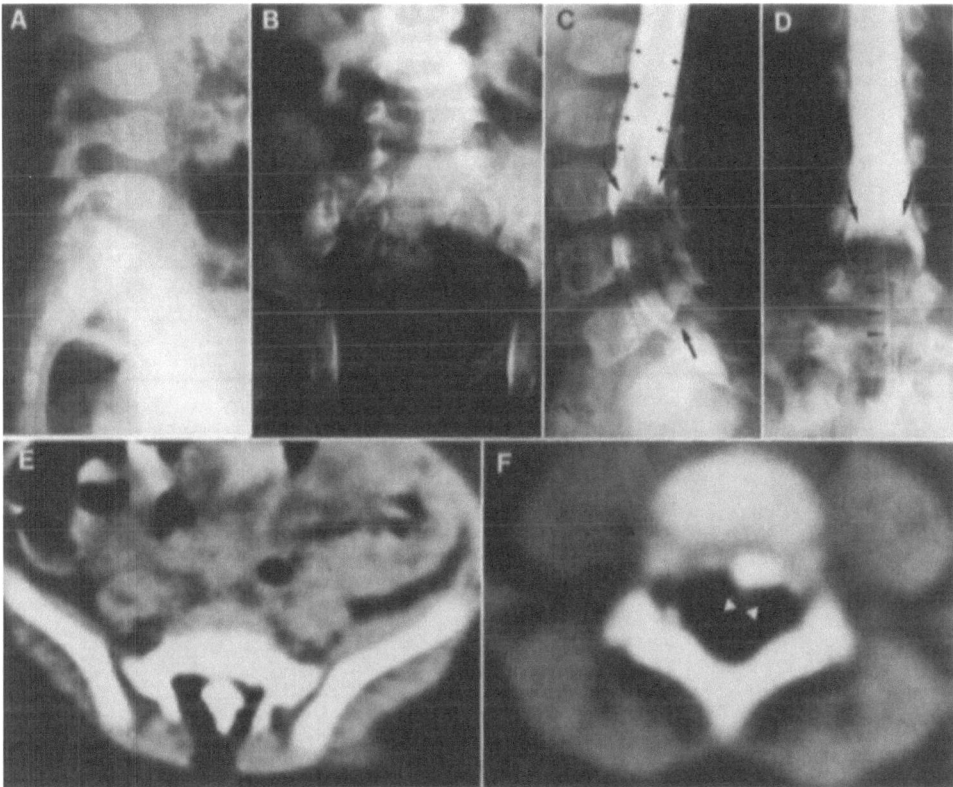

Figure 3.7. Lypoma and tethered cord. **A,B** Plain x-ray films show scalloping of the posterior vertebral bodies of L-3 and L-4 as well as lumbosacral rachischisis. **C,D** At myelography there is an obvious tethered cord (*small arrows*) ending in an intradural ovoid mass (*large arrows*). In **D** a thin line of contrast medium splits the mass (*arrowheads*). **E,F** Myelo-Ct demonstrates the low-density lipoma with its extradural (**E**) and intradural (**F**) component. In **E** the tethered cord appears infiltrated by the fatty tissue, and there is a curious "heart shaped" axial configuration because of the above-mentioned opacified CSF split (*arrowheads*).

6 months of life, US is restricted to the evaluation of spinal malformations (above all spina bifida) and of the associated "maldevelopmental tumors" (20,76). Furthermore, US has recently been introduced as an intraoperative guide in spinal cord surgery (88,89). The use of intraoperative spinal US appears particularly significant in guiding the resection of intramedullary tumors; in these cases US easily differentiates solid neoplastic nodules from the accompanying cystic dilation of the central canal and monitors the progressive and precise excision of the lesions (90).

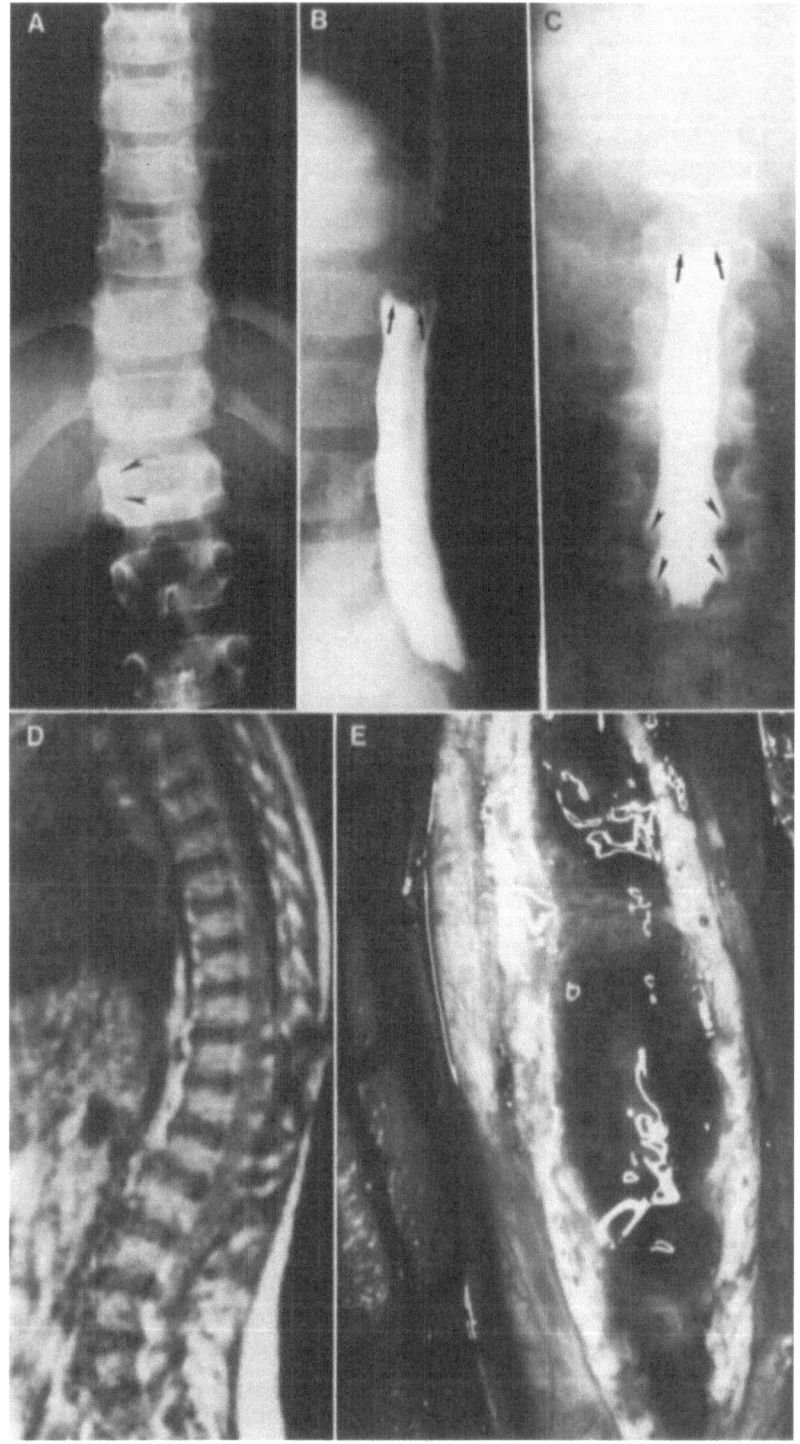

Myelography

The availability of the new and safer nonionic water-soluble contrast media (metrizamide, iopamidol, ioexol) has ruled out the risk of late arachnoiditis, which was often encountered with oil myelography. Despite this clear advantage, the use of myelography in spinal diagnoses has been slowly declining since the introduction of the modern imaging techniques. Generally speaking, invasive intrathecal contrast studies will more than likely be abolished in the near future. Today, however, myelography is the most basic step in pediatric spinal diagnosis due to the limited availability of MRI and to the residual technical problems in pediatric MRI studies (see below).

Careful myelographic evaluation demonstrates both the normal anatomy of the spinal cord, roots, and subarachnoid spaces and the site and extension of the spinal tumors. In most cases conventional myelographic semiotics is able to define the relationship between a spinal mass, the dural coverings, and the spinal cord, thus identifying extradural, intradural, extramedullary, and intramedullary lesions (38,54,100). Usually, this diagnosis is possible also when the tumor completely blocks the subarachnoid spaces. In such a condition, however, myelography cannot show the upper pole of the tumor without a further introduction of contrast medium above the block, usually by the laterocervical route. Today this procedure appears to be not only of no use but also an additional risk in most patients because CT following myelography (so called "myelo-CT") usually succeeds in demonstrating the minimal amounts of contrast medium above the block, thus defining the cranial pole of the lesion (29,53) (Fig. 3.9). Generally speaking, myelographic blocks, as well as any positive or equivocal myelography, must be completed by myelo-CT; in fact, the additional information provided by intrathecally enhanced CT is an invaluable advantage (see below, CT).

Computed Tomography

All modern CT equipment provides the basic capabilities required for a complete spinal pediatric examination. In fact, scout views, high-resolution

◁────────────────────────────────────

Figure 3.8. Ependymoma of the conus medullaris in a 9-year-old boy. **A** Standard AP film of the spine reveals scoliosis and minimal thinning (*arrowheads*) of the right L-1 pedicle. **B,C** Myelography demonstrates an intradural-obstructing tumor with its lower pole at L-2 (*arrows*). There is mild ectasia of the lumbosacral dural sac and root sleeves (*arrowheads*). At surgery complete excision of the ependymoma was performed. **D** Two years after the operation, the patient experienced recurrence of the painful symptoms. MRI (sagittal proton-density image) discloses a recurrent hypointense expansive lesion extending from the conus to D-7 vertebral body. **E** At the operation, a recurrent intramedullary tumor is exposed by multiple laminectomy. The tumor was again apparently removed totally without neurological deficits.

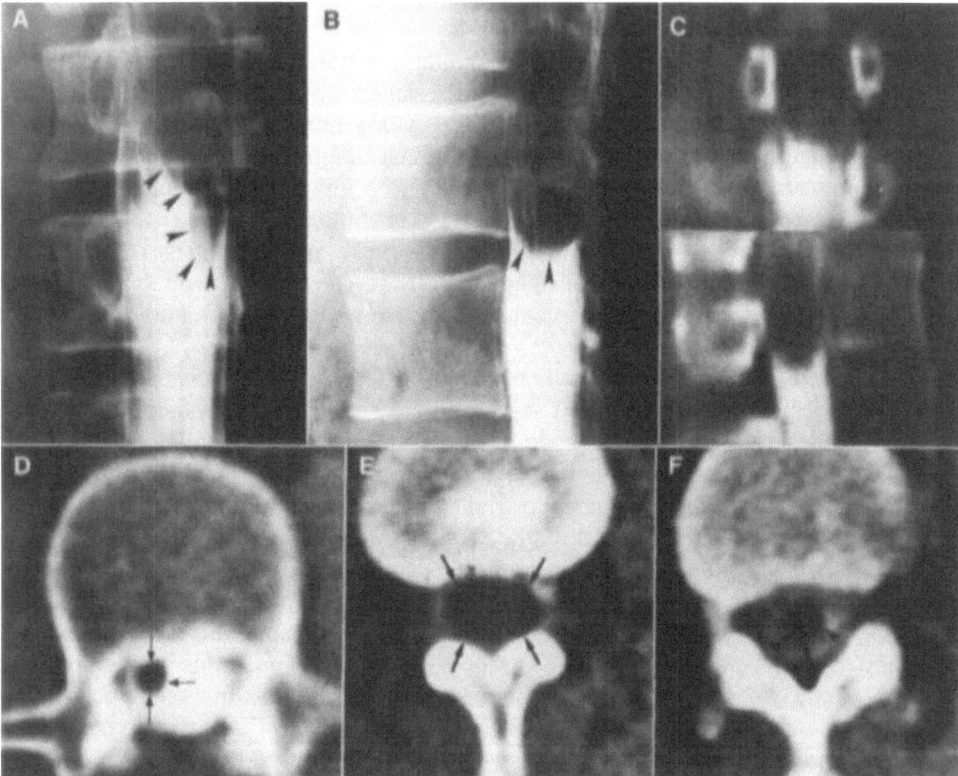

Figure 3.9. Dermoid of the conus medullaris. Myelography reveals an intradural mass but fails to demonstrate its intramedullary or extramedullary location because of the complete myelographic block. Myelo-CT demonstrates the medullary location of the lesion by means of its superior contrast resolution. **A,B** Conventional myelograms outline the lower lobulated pole (*arrowheads*) of the intradural mass lesion, resulting in a complete block. **C** Coronal and sagittal reformatted images reveal minimal amount of contrast medium above the tumor, outlining its superior pole. **D–F** Contiguous axial slices depict the shape of the hypodense tumor (*arrows*) and the normally positioned conus medullaris (*arrowheads* in **F**), so demonstrating the intramedullary location of the lesion.

algorhithms, target and zoom reconstruction, and multiplanar reformation of the axial slices are now available in all equipment and represent a great technical improvement, resulting in a more precise and definite diagnosis.

When clinical and radiological findings suggest a spinal cord (or root) compression, and MRI is not available, intrathecally enhanced CT (myelo-CT) is probably the method of choice. Myelo-CT in most cases is performed after conventional myelograms (secondary myelo-CT); but when there is a precise (clinical or radiologic) localization of the area of interest, one may avoid preliminary myelography because primary myelo-CT re-

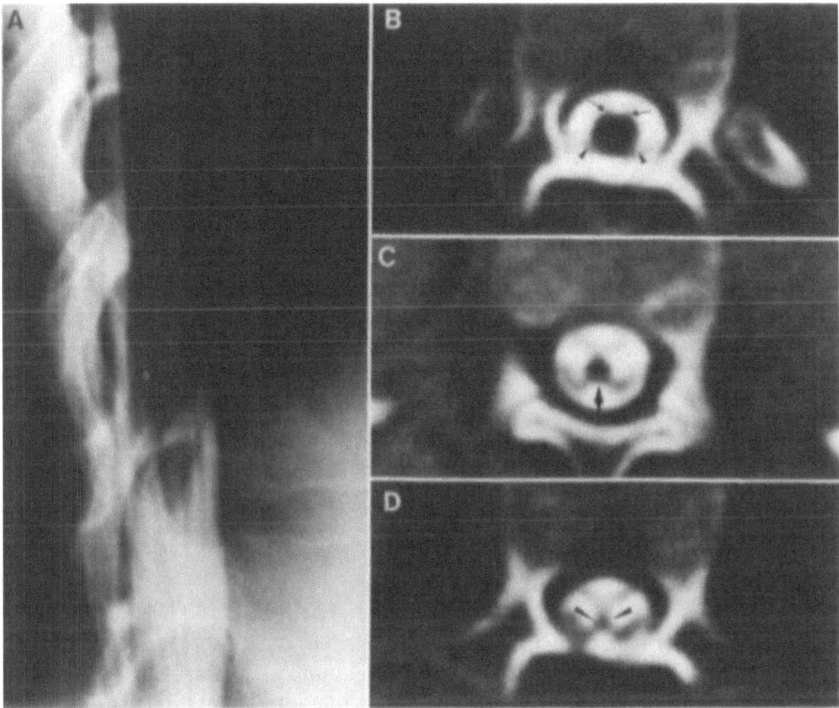

Figure 3.10. Myelo-CT depicting normal anatomy of the conus medullaris and filum terminale in a 4-year-old child. **A** Myelogram, lateral view. **B** Conus medullaris with anterior (*arrows*) and posterior roots (*arrowheads*). **C** Tip of the conus medullaris (*large arrow*) with roots. **D** Central filum terminale (*arrowheads*) with X-shaped appearance of the root of the cauda equina.

quires a much smaller amount of contrast medium and the possible adverse reactions are less frequent and less severe (53). In children the intrathecal introduction of 2 to 3 ml of isotonic (150 to 180 mg/mL of iodine) nonionic water-soluble contrast medium provides an optimal picture of cross-sectional and multiplanar anatomy of the spinal cord, subarachnoid spaces, and spinal canal (Figs. 3.10, 3.11). Myelo-CT, unlike myelography, gives further significant information about the density of the lesions and their possible extraspinal extension. Low-density lipomas (Fig. 3.7) are easily identified by CT, also, a minimal deposition of calcium within a soft-tissue lesion can be imaged by CT when its density is not enough to be detected by conventional radiographic studies. When there is an extraspinal extension, the examination may be further completed by intravenous contrast enhancement to improve the visualization of richly vascularized lesions (Fig. 3.5), detect areas of necrosis, and disclose possible invasion of critical blood vessels (i.e., aorta or vena cava) (29). As previously mentioned,

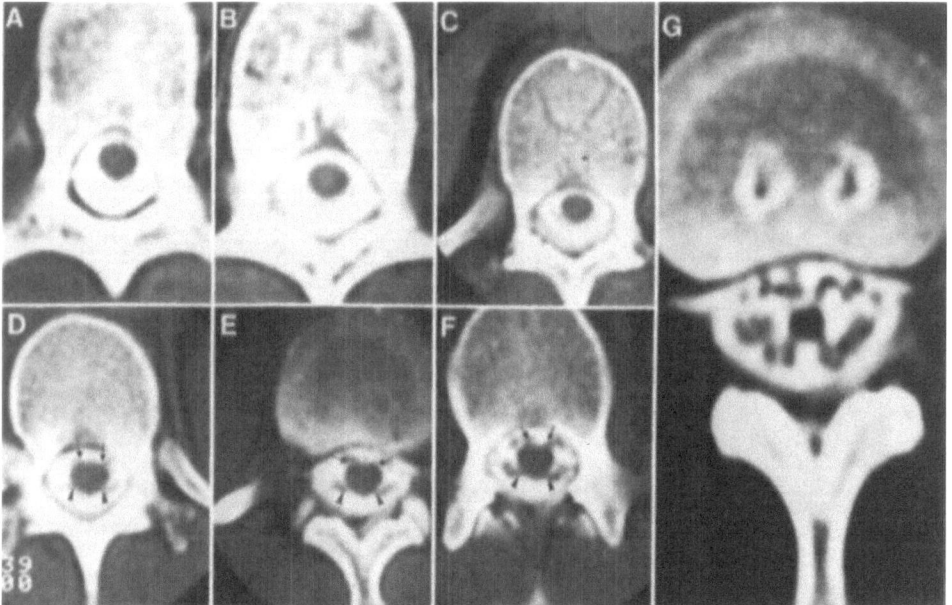

Figure 3.11. Normal anatomy (in a 14-year-old girl) of the lower dorsal spinal cord with conus medullaris and roots of the cauda equina, as demonstrted by myelo-CT. **A–C** Normal lower thoracic cord occupies the anterior part of the opacified thecal sac. **D–F** Normal conus medullaris with anterior (*arrows*) and posterior (*arrowheads*) merging roots. **G** At the level of the tip of the conus medullaris the roots of the cauda equina are arranged in regular X-shaped configurations.

myelo-CT is mandatory when a complete block is demonstrated by myelography. The superior contrast resolution of CT may, in most cases, visualize the upper extension of the obstructing lesion. Furthermore, in some instances (especially in the region of the conus medullaris/cauda equina) myelo-CT succeeds in defining the correct source of an obstructing intradural tumor (intramedullary or extramedullary) when this definition is not possible at myelography (Fig. 3.9). In patients with suspected intramedullary cavitation, serial CT studies must be obtained at least 6 and 20 hours after intrathecal introduction of the contrast medium because of the possible subsequent opacification of the "cysts."

Sometimes, when clinical symptoms and/or previous radiographic findings suggest a bony spinal abnormality or a purely paraspinal tumor, without involvement of the intraspinal structures, a satisfactory depiction of the lesion is obtained only by intravenously enhanced CT (IVECT). Also, IVECT is sufficient in cases where one must control a known extramedullary tumor that had disclosed a strong contrast uptake in a previous examination. Despite some exceptions (63), an intraspinal tumor cannot be ruled out by means of IVECT.

Magnetic Resonance Imaging

The MRI is a revolutionary and more frequently used modality for imaging and tissue characterization that promises to replace all other radiological methods and techniques in neuroradiology (11,24,60). Briefly, MRI is based on modifications induced in the human body (placed in a high-magnetic stationary field) when appropriate radiofrequencies (RF) are applied. Such modifications in the state of energy of the body components result in a RF signal that is received by specialized antennas (coils) and then measured and computed. The transformation of the RF signals into anatomical images is obtained by computerized processes almost similar to those used in CT. Thus, the depiction of an anatomical slice results from the digital, numerical, and computerized representation of several physical properties. In CT the basic physical property influencing the images is the density or, in other words, the attenuation of the x-ray beams. On the other hand, in MRI the basic physical properties are several and more complex (11). The MR signal received in any pixel is a function of three basic parameters of the corresponding point of the sample: proton density (density of the spins) and relaxation times T1 and T2 (T1-longitudinal relaxation time; T2-transverse relaxation time). Furthermore, the presence of the flow also influences the signal intensity. In practice, MRI reflects the magnetic behavior and density of the hydrogen protons.

Unlike CT, MRI is a multiparametric modality of imaging and tissue characterization, and such multiple parameters give rise to the wide capabilities and potential development of the method. The clear advantages of MRI, in comparison with other imaging methods are (a) absence of radiation exposure and no need of a hazardous contrast medium, (b) superior soft-tissue contrast and resolution, and (c) direct multiplanar images in any desired plane of the proper mode of imaging (so-called sequences). The most common and useful mode of imaging is the spin echo (SE) sequence in which one can select the parameters of repetition time (TR) and echo times (TE) in turn. By selecting TR and TE it is possible to obtain images (and signal intensities) influenced mainly by proton density, T1, or T2. To simplify this concept one can assume that SE sequences with short TR and short TE are mainly a function of T1 ("T1 weighted"), whereas the use of long TR and long TE makes the images primarily dependent on T2 ("T2 weighted"). Using long TR and short TE it is possible to minimize the effects of both T1 and T2, thus obtaining images and signal intensities that reflect proton density.

Magnetic resonance imaging has a main overall disadvantage: the tremendous cost of the equipment and, therefore, a relatively limited availability. In the pediatric population there is another important disadvantage arising from the need for absolute immobility of the patient being examined for long periods of time (generally from 30 to 60 minutes) (12). Thus, heavy sedation is required in all younger and uncooperative children, and, moreover, patient monitoring is problematic in the MRI rooms because of the hazard of introducing ferromagnetic objects and the serious dysfunction of the monitoring equipment when introduced into the high magnetic field.

The use of proper coils represents a basic point in spinal MRI (73); the cervical spine can be examined by conventional head coils whereas the use of specialized "surface" coils is mandatory in the evaluation of thoracic and lumbar spines. By means of surface coils, improvement in image quality is dramatic, resulting from the short distance between the area of interest and the receiver coil (increased signal-to-noise ratio).

In general, when using surface coils and T1-weighted images, morphological studies with fine anatomical details are obtained; use of the progressively T2-weighted images, and comparison with the T1-weighted images, gives a tissue characterization. In T1-weighted images of the spine (Figs. 3.12, 3.13A), the CSF has a low intensity (black), the spinal cord has a higher signal (gray), and the epidural fat exibits the highest intensity (white). The behavior of the bony structures (i.e., vertebrae) is different

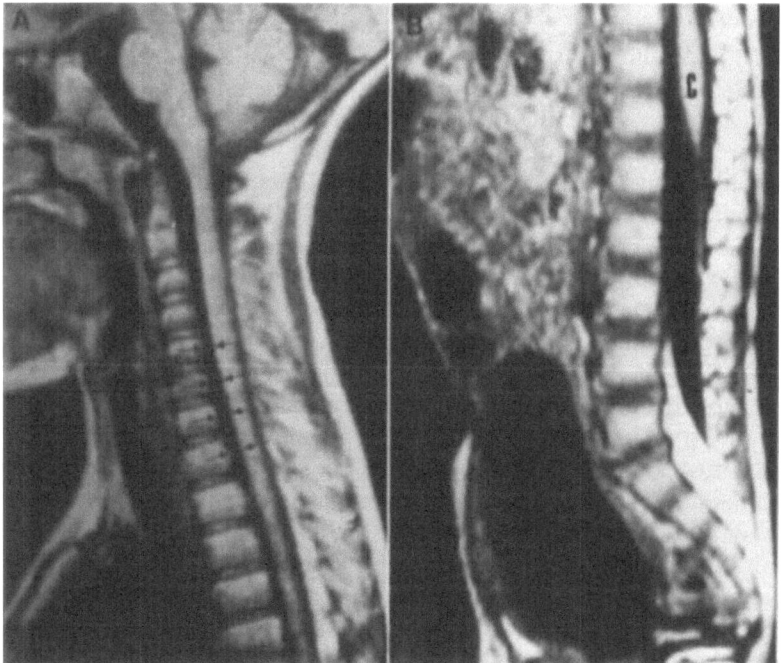

Figure 3.12. Normal sagittal T1-weighted MRIs of the craniocervical and upper dorsal spine (**A**) and of the lumbosacral spine (**B**). Fine anatomical details are obtained in the lumbosacral area by means of the surface coils and T1-weighted images (see text). In **A** there is good morphological demonstration of the cervicomedullary junction; note the wide black space between the posterior surface of the cervical vertebral bodies and the cord (*arrows*). This space reflects the absence of signal from cortical bone. In **B** the conus medullaris (**C**) with its tip is perfectly visualized.

for cancellous bone and cortical bone: the former appears intense, similar to muscles and other parenchyma, whereas the latter is black (because of poor signals arising from the "fixed" protons), and it is not easy to separate from the adjacent CSF in the subarachnoid spaces. This situation explains the apparently wide space that is visible in sagittal T1 images between the spinal cord and the signal of the posterior vertebral body. In the heavily weighted T2 images there is a clear-cut change in the observed

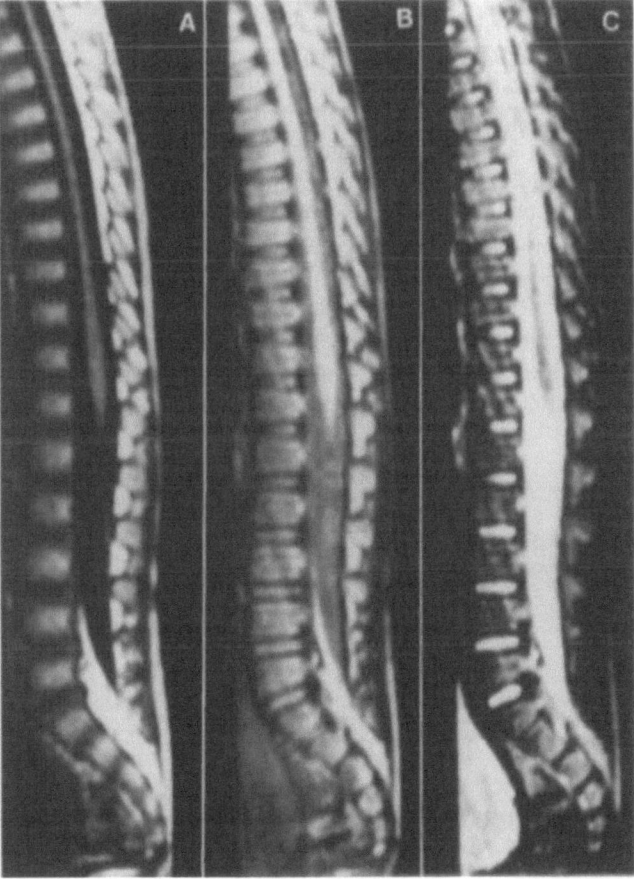

Figure 3.13. MRI of the normal dorsolumbar spine in childhood (4-year-old boy). Modifications of the signal intensities upon different weighting of the spin echo sequences (see also test). **A** In the sagittal T1-weighted image, subarachnoid CSF has low intensity (black), epidural fat (dots), high intensity (white), spinal cord intermediate intensity (gray). **B** In the moderately T2-weighted image there is a slight increase in the CSF intensity (which becomes gray). **C** In the heavily T2-weighted image CSF in the subarachnoid spaces is markedly hyperintense (white) while spinal cord exhibits low intensity (dark gray). Consequently the picture resembles the myelogram (the so-called "myelographic effect" in T2-MRI).

intensity (Figs. 3.13B, 3.13C): the CSF becomes hyperintense (white) because of its very long T2, while all other structures lose intensity, becoming darker than the CSF. This behavior makes the images somewhat similar to those of myelography and maximizes the evidence of any subarachnoid space encroachment (thus justifying the term "myelographic effect" used to describe these heavily weighted T2 images).

Before concluding this simplified approach to spinal MRI, it is useful to underline some general features about the pathological modifications of the signal (80).

1. Most of the tumors (and other pathologies) show an increase in both T1 and T2 values (in comparison with those of normal nervous tissue), resulting in a hypointensity in the T1-weighted images and in a hyperintensity in the T2-weighted images. This common behavior explains the low specificity of the method and, for example, the difficult differentiation between the tumors and the surrounding edema.
2. In general, liquid-containing cavities exhibit an intensity directly related to their protein content. Therefore, whereas simple hydromyelic or syringomyelic "cysts" contain pure CSF with a low protein content and a very weak signal (black), cysts within a tumor show slightly higher signals (gray) because of their higher proteinaceous content.
3. Fat tissue, and therefore lipomas as well (Fig. 3.14), has a high intensity

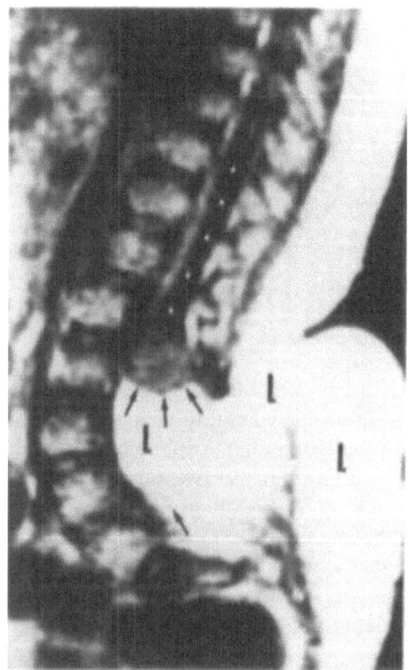

Figure 3.14. Lipomeningomyelocele with tethered cord and hydromyelia. In this sagittal T1-weighted MRI the subcutaneous and intraspinal lipoma is easily demonstrated with typical hyperintensity (L). Note the placode (*arrows*) and the dilatation of the central canal because of hydromyelia (*white points*).

(it looks white) in the T1-weighted images (because of their very short T1 value).

4. The subacute hematomas are also hyperintense in T1-weighted images because of the large amount of methemoglobin.

5. Rapid or strong flowing liquids exhibit extremely low signals (dark black) in all sequences because of the flowing away of the excited protons. This phenomenon, known as the "flow void sign," facilitates the recognition of the larger blood vessels and may suggest the presence of a vascular malformation.

6. In all sequences calcifications also appear black (weak signal) because of the limited "mobility" of their proton content (as in cortical bones). Unfortunately, minimal calcium deposits are not easy to distinguish, and, in general, MRI is less sensitive than CT in this field.

Angiography

Indications for a selective study of the spinal vascularization are myelographic, CT, or MRI evidence of abnormal blood vessels in the spine and spinal cord, suggesting a vascular malformation or a richly vascularized tumor. In both instances an angiographic diagnosis may be the first step in the interventional angiographic procedure. Surgical neuroangiographic methods allow the complete treatment of spinal vascular malformations, or they may be followed by the subsequent surgical excision of residual abnormalities. In many cases of nonresectable, pain-producing spinal tumors, interventional radiology also obtains goods palliative results. In every case the aim of endovascular radiological treatment is devascularization (complete if possible) of the lesions without interfering with the critical blood vessels supplying the spinal cord (27,94). Today, a wide variety of liquids, particles, and balloons are available to obtain a successful embolization and devascularization of any kind of lesion.

An up-to-date protocol for the neuroradiological evaluation of suspected spinal tumors may be suggested after this concise review of the methods and their possibilities. In 1981 Harwood-Nash (53) proposed a neuroradiological approach to the diagnosis of spinal diseases; his protocol was based on the results of the preliminary plain films of the spine and was clearly influenced by the increasing capabilities resulting from the use of CT and myelo-CT. Within the last few years, however, the introduction of MRI has replaced CT as the main diagnostic modality. Thus, the Harwood-Nash protocol may be modified as follows, provided the MRI equipment is available:

When there is any X-ray sign of an intraspinal expansile lesion, MRI should follow to confirm or rule out an intraspinal tumor. Also, in cases in which there is strong clinical suspicion of an intraspinal tumor even without any conventional radiographic finding, MRI is the method of choice. If MRI definitely excludes the presence of a tumor or, on the contrary, clearly demonstrates and characterizes such a lesion, the flow chart stops. In such instances the combination "standard X-ray + MRI" gives all the necessary information to select the correct treatment in most cases. Only selected cases require further conventional evaluation by means of myelo-CT.

In the presence of conventional radiographic evidence of acquired bony (vertebral) structural changes in a child, RNS are probably indicated to exclude more extensive pathology (e.g., multiple lesions in histiocytosis X, leukemia, multiple sarcomatous metastasis). Then, provided the presence of a solitary bony lesion is ascertained, CT may be the proper method of evaluation using the myelo-CT technique or, in selected cases only, intravenous enhancement (see above, CT). The satisfactory CT delineation of both soft and bony tissues so far seems to justify the use of CT instead of MRI in bone tumors.

In patients with X-ray evidence of spina bifida, the method of choice is myelo-CT because the better spatial resolution allows the demonstration of subtle structures like the filum terminalis and the roots. High-resolution US represents a satisfactory noninvasive alternative for studying these patients. However, in many pediatric patients with maldevelopmental tumors accompanying spina bifida, MRI becomes necessary; for example, to disclose Chiari II malformation or associated syringo-hydro-myelia (Fig. 3.14) (9). In all instances in which MRI is not available, the use of myelo-CT becomes mandatory.

The technology of MRI appears to be increasing and spreading so rapidly that in the near future the statement "MRI, the single method of imaging the spine" will not appear exaggerated.

Extramedullary Tumors

Maldevelopmental Tumors

This group includes several types of histologically benign lesions frequently associated with spinal dysraphia. Three main categories can be schematically distinguished: Dysgenetic tumors containing derivatives of the primitive cell layers (epidermoids and dermoids, teratomas, neurenteric cysts), ectopic hamartomas of the meninges and sacrum (chordomas, ectopic ependymomas), and dysplastic tumors, such as those occurring in cases of neuroectodermal blastomatosis (e.g., the tumors associated with Recklinghausen's disease). However, only a limited variety of pathological forms have clinical relevance in children and will be dealt with in this chapter.

Dysgenetic Tumors

These tumors originate from inclusions deriving from the three primitive cell layers (Fig. 3.15). The *epidermoids,* consisting of a simple epidermal structure surrounding cholesterine deposits, originate from the ectoderm,

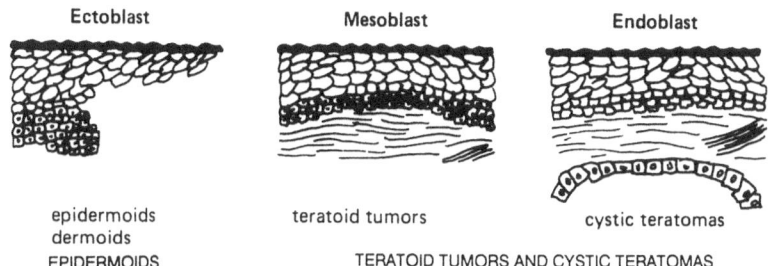

Figure 3.15. Schematic drawing illustrating the origin of the dysgenetic tumors from inclusions of the three primitive cell layers (see text).

as do the *dermoids,* which are characterized by a dermal-epidermal structure, including hairs and sebaceous glands. These tumors appear in nearly all age groups, with equal distribution both in children and adults (112), i.e., around 12% to 14% of all the vertebro-medullary tumors. Typical locations are in the lumbar and lumbosacral areas, with a higher incidence at the conus.

The possible causative role of repeated lumbar spinal punctures in the genesis of epidermoid and dermoid tumors was first proposed by Choremis and co-workers in 1956 (16) and subsequently supported by several authors (10,67,101). The etiopathogenetic mechanism was identified in infants receiving spinal needles without a stylet inserted, which facilitates the penetration of skin fragments and their subsequent growth within the spinal cord and surrounding subarachnoid space (16,41). This hypothesis was also confirmed by experimental observations of epidermoids and dermoids developing in the rat from simple pieces of skin placed within and adjacent to the subarachnoid spinal space shortly after birth (111).

In most instances these tumors are intradural and extramedullary, with the possible exception of those developing in the conus and cauda equina regions, which may be extra/intramedullary at the same time. These lesions are rarely confined completely within the spinal cord or the extradural space.

In most cases dermoids or epidermoids show only minimal abnormalities in the spine X-ray films, usually a small increase in the interpedunculate distance and a thinning of the pedicles (sometimes associated with posterior rachischisis).

Myelography and myelo-CT (Figs. 3.9, 3.16) are commonly used for diagnosis delineating the mass within the subarachnoid space or with the spinal cord. When the mass completely occupies the dural sac in the region of the conus medullaris, obstructing the subarachnoid spaces, only myelo-CT is able to define the intra or extramedullary site of these mass lesions. Usually, both dermoids and epidermoids exhibit low attenuation value (hypodense lesions) (29,75).

Teratomas have a more complex structure than that of dermoids and epidermoids, as they originate from remnants of two or all three embryonic

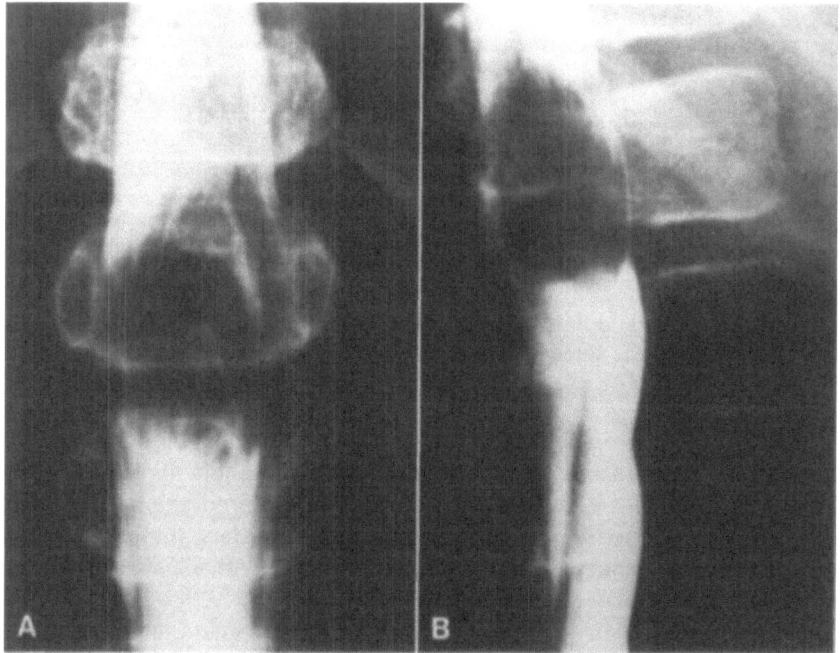

Figure 3.16. Dermoid of the conus medullaris. **A,B** Myelography outlines the intradural mass that expands the conus.

layers and may include differentiated connective tissues (muscle, bone, cartilage) as well as parenchymal tissues (lung, thyroid) (112). Two main forms may be distinguished: the solid form—teratoid tumors—from the mesoblast, and the cystic form—cystic teratomas—from the endoblast. The sacrococcygeal region and the intradural space are the most common locations. Teratoid tumors, however, also frequently occupy the cervicodorsal region. Teratomas are generally recognized at a younger age (about 4 years) than epidermoids and dermoids (about 8 years) (112). The presence of an associated dermal sinus may facilitate the early recognition of either dermoids and epidermoids or teratomas. This association may account for the principal complication of these types of tumor, i.e., meningeal infections through the sinus tract. However, meningeal signs may occasionally be related directly to the irritant effect of the cystic content of the tumor (21).

The duration of symptoms varies greatly from weeks to years, with the teratoid tumors becoming noticeable earlier than the epidermoids or dermoids. The onset of clinical symptoms is characterized, in order of frequency, by spine and radicular pain, static disturbances, and pseudoabdominal signs (112). When the symptoms are fully established, a stiffness of the spine, often associated with scoliosis, kyphosis, or hyperlordosis, is the most common sign together with paraparesis. Motor deficits are usually spastic and bilateral, although a unilateral weakness may be encountered in about a third of the children. Tetraparesis may correspond to the presence of a teratoid tumor in the cervical region. Flaccid paralyses occur in less than a fourth of the cases. Sphincter disturbances are common when the lesion is fully established.

In the most frequently encountered sacrococcygeal location, teratomas result in various degrees of radiological findings. In some instances spine X-ray findings are almost normal, with only the soft-tissue mass demonstrated; in other cases there are signs of expanding intraspinal mass or, more frequently, agenesis of lower coccygeal vertebral elements. In every case CT is the method of choice, characterizing both the exact relationships of the mass and the cystic/solid components (Fig. 3.17). Ultrasonography is also indicated in these patients, with similar capabilities.

In about half the cases, plain spine X-ray films demonstrate abnormalities such as an increased interpeduncular distance, posterior erosion of one or more vertebrae, and erosion of one pedicle, as well as congenital anomalies, namely, spina bifida occulta (104).

Treatment of epidermoids, dermoids, and teratomas consists in removing the intraspinal cystic tumor and, when present, the associated sinus tract. Removal is usually total and without neurological damage in cases of extramedullary lesions. Generally, epidermoids, dermoids, and teratoid tumors can be totally excised, whereas cystic teratomas are often incompletely removed and may require multiple surgical procedures.

Neurenteric Cysts

First described by Keen and Coplin in 1906 (58), these cysts are thought to arise from persistence of the neurenteric accessory canal or from entodermal remnants that have not been separated from the notochord by mesodermal cells (28). They appear macroscopically as cystic lesions of the spinal axis connected at a distance with the digestive tract. A neurenteric cyst, known under such different terms as gastrocytoma, teratoma cyst, or mediastinal cyst of the primitive digestive system, may develop either intradurally or extradurally and preferably at the dorsal level. Histologically, they are usually lined by a cuboidal or mucus-secreting epithelium, resembling that of the esophagus or, less frequently, the stomach. In other cases these cysts have a structure comparable to that of the respiratory airways (17). Respiratory or digestive symptoms or signs of spinal cord compression usually reveal the lesion. The radiological demonstration of a vertebral defect in the anterior spinal canal wall is of particular importance for the diagnosis. However, bone anomalies may be lacking in some subjects, as neurenteric cysts exclusively confined within the spinal canal have been described (17). An accurate pelvic examination, barium enema, or contrast medium examination of the digestive system may provide important diagnostic findings. The excision of this type of lesion usu-

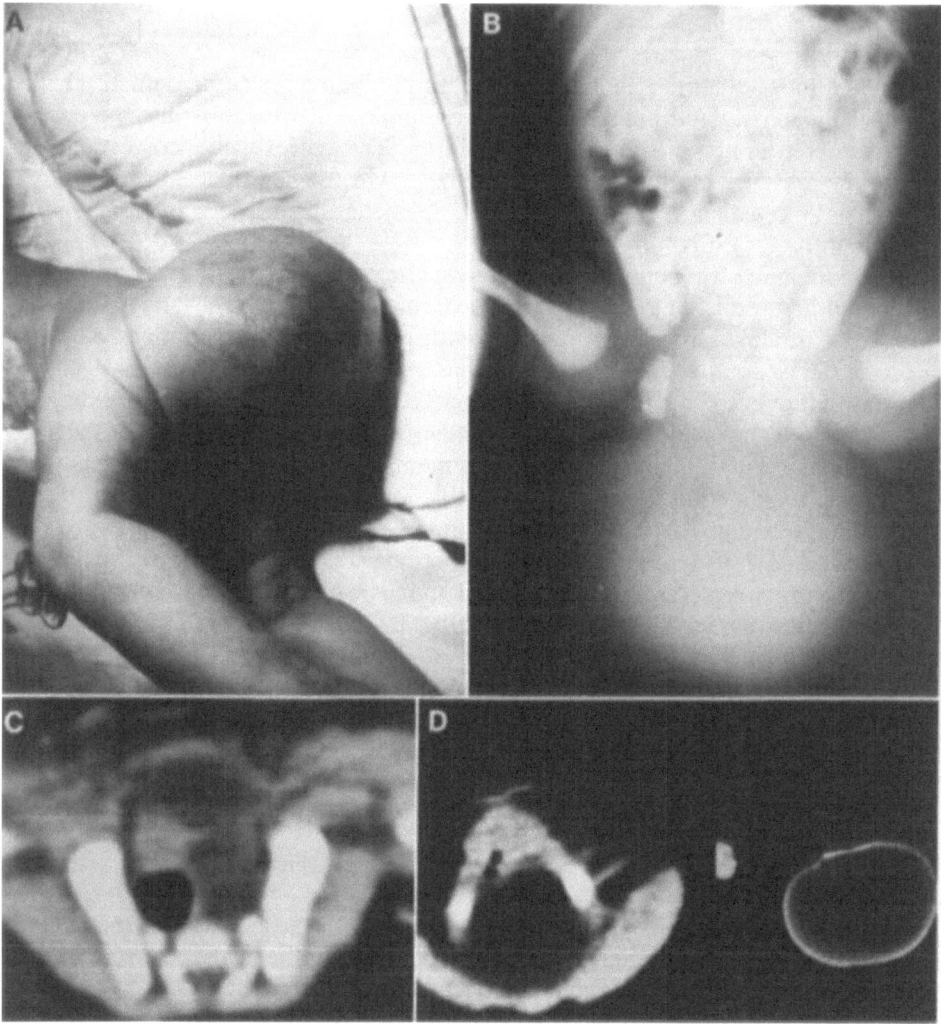

Figure 3.17. Cystic coccygeal teratoma in a newborn. **A** Clinical presentation of the huge mass. **B** Standard x-ray study shows soft-tissue density of the mass without calcium deposits. Caudal coccygeal vertebrae are lacking. **C,D** Computed tomography. *Axial* unenhanced slices confirm the liquid-containing mass.

ally requires two separate approaches in order to remove the intraspinal component and the extraspinal mass.

Lipomas

Lipomas are relatively common in children in association with rachischisis. However, they can occur, even though rarely, as discrete intradural extramedullary lesions, which may evolve without symptoms for a long time, and in persons without any evidence of a neural tube defect (26). Also, in these cases associated cutaneous anomalies such as subcutaneous masses or dimples are relatively common (Fig. 3.18) (64). The entire region

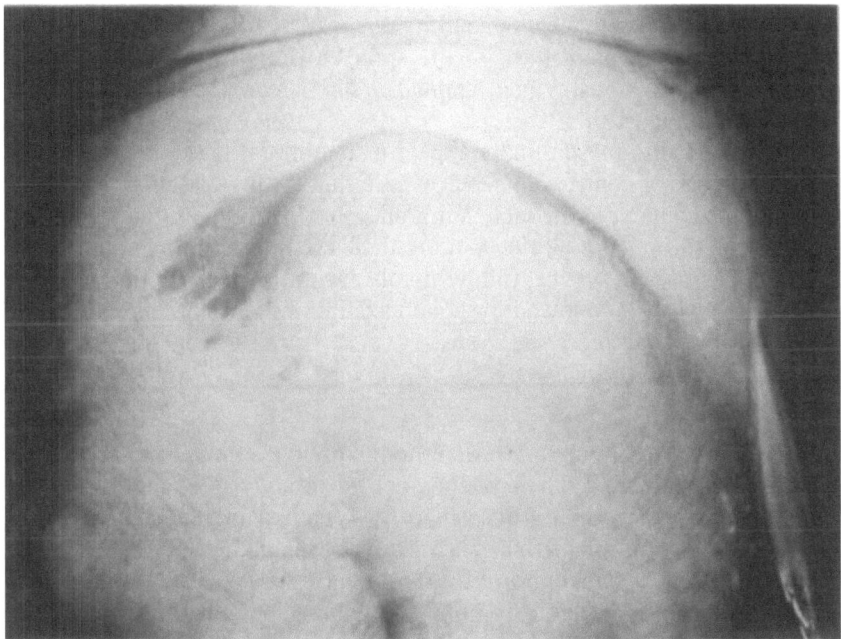

Figure 3.18. Asymmetric low back mass of a lipoma; note also the pigmented skin.

of the spine may be involved, although most of these lesions are found in anatomical relationship to the conus, filum terminalis, and cauda equina roots. In symptomatic cases the most common initial complaint is a slowly ascending monoparesis or paraparesis. Sphincter disturbances are also frequent. Pain is characteristically absent on the whole, even in subjects showing radiological evidence of an expanding intraspinal mass.

All neuroradiological methods are commonly used in the diagnosis of spinal lipomas: plain spine x-ray, US, myelo-CT, and MRI all may contribute to the optimal evaluation of these maldevelopmental tumors. When there is a meningomyelocele, or an obvious lipomemingomyelocele, the child is usually evaluated in the neonatal period and the first approach is probably a combination of standard films of the spine and high-resolution US, which results in delineating the content of the low back mass and the associated tethered cord (76,89). However, myelo-CT and MRI appear to be the method of choice when the surgeon needs to know the precise relationship between the lipoma, the tethered cord (Fig. 3.7), and the roots of the cauda equina. This also applies in cases where the patients are observed at a later age or after previous resection of the meningomyelocele (75).

The very low attenuation values of the lipomas make the diagnosis easy by means of CT, but the recognition of such lesions is also obvious by means of MRI because of the nearly pathognomonic hyperintensity in the T1-weighted images (short T1) (80). Thus, when a lipoma is suspected (without meningomyeloceles or cutaneous signs), MRI should follow directly the standard plain films of the spine. Moreover, MRI has the advantage of disclosing associated anomalies like Chiari II malformation and hydromyelia (Fig. 3.14).

Macroscopically, these tumors appear as mature fat tissue provided with a wide network of connective septa, where fine-feeding vascular structures run. Lipomas appear as strongly adherent to or in direct continuation with the nervous tissue (Fig. 3.19), making their complete removal almost always impossible. However, follow-up observations indicate that subtotal or partial excision is followed by a stabilization in neurological conditions. Radiotherapy is ineffective.

Chordomas

These tumors are rare in children, although they are thought to arise from notochordal remnants. Their occurrence in infancy is exceptional (81). Chordomas were originally described by Luschka in 1856, but the first histological description of this type of tumor was made by Virchow, who coined the term "physaliphorous" to indicate the large vacuolated cells typical of this lesion. The resemblance of these cells to those of the notochord was noted by Muller two years after Luschka's description. At the end of the 19th century, Ribbert obtained a tumor resembling the

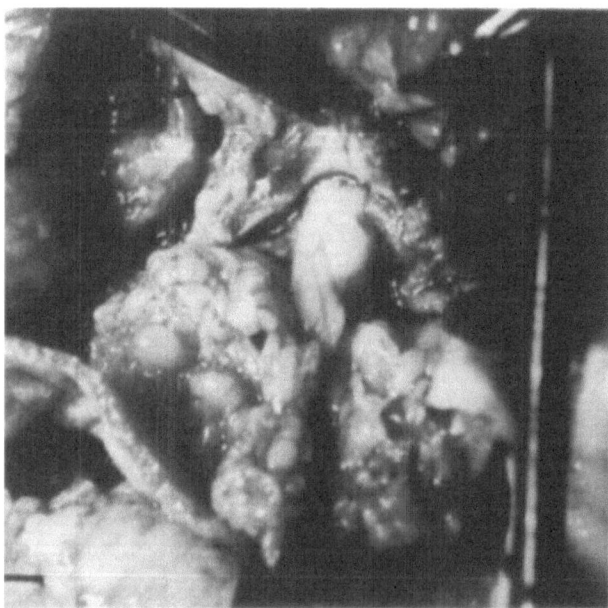

Figure 3.19. Intraoperative view of the lobulated surface of a lipoma intimately adherent to the tethered cord.

chordoma by puncturing the intervertebral disk in the rabbit. More recently, electron microscopic observations have further confirmed the similarity between chordomas and the nucleus polposus of the intervertebral disk (74,83). Although histologically benign, these tumors, which are formed of a myxoid tissue, behave as a malignant and sometimes very aggressive lesion. Recurrences are constant and metastases possible.

The onset of clinical manifestations in children is marked by pain and stiffness of the spine. In the initial phase the plain X-ray examination may remain negative. The symptomatology subsequently evolves, with the signs of a pharyngeal tumor in cases of an anterior growth of the tumor from the clivus, or compression of the spinal cord or cauda equina roots in cases of a prevalently intraspinal development. When the chordoma grows cephalad (cranially), the clinical picture may be consistent with that of a posterior cranial fossa expanding mass. When the lesion is advanced, areas of osteolysis or bone hyperdensity may be demonstrated at the radiological examination. The presence of chordomas is typically characterized by destructive changes in the vertebral body, with involvement of the discal space (36), and by a prevertebral soft mass (which on CT scans appears to have the same density as muscles). This latter examination may also reveal a variable degree of calcification associated with the osseous destruction induced by the tumor in more than half the patients.

Surgical resection and radiotherapy are the two main therapeutic possibilities in the treatment of chordomas, but results are unfavorable in the large majority of patients, even when the two types of treatment are combined. Macroscopically, the tumor appears well demarcated and lobulated, with a pseudocapsule limiting the soft component but without any apparent capsule separating it from the bone. Infiltration of paravertebral structures is possible, especially in recurrent cases. In the sacrococcygeal location, gross excision of the mass may be aided by a double approach to the sacrum and to the intraabdominal component of the tumor. Conversely, removal of the vertebral lesion is less rewarding because of the usually large epidural extension at the time of the diagnosis. In some advanced cases, surgery may be limited to a decompressive procedure performed through a posterior laminectomy.

Although chordomas are radioresistant tumors, external radiation therapy is usually performed for palliative purposes in inoperable subjects using techniques that allow effective treatment of the tumor while sparing the healthy spinal cord and radicular structures. Interstitial radiotherapy using [192]iridium and proton beam therapy have also been proposed (108). Chemotherapy has invariably proved to be unsuccessful.

Ectopic Ependymomas

These tumors originate from ependymal cells in heterotopic positions, such as within the coccygeal ligament, or in extraspinal positions. They should be distinguished from the more common ependymomas related to ependymal cell clusters of the filum terminale. Three main pathogenetic explanations have been proposed. According to the first one, these tumors originate from the coccygeal medullary vestige, which is an ependymal-lined cavity in the caudal portion of the neural tube beneath the skin of the postnatal pit (96). Such an explanation, however, accounts for only those ectopic ependymomas localized in the coccygeal region and developing as a soft-tissue mass, either posteriorly to the sacrum, or anteriorly in the retro-rectal space of the pelvis. A second explanation postulates that remnants of the neurenteric canal give origin to nervous cells in the sacral area and paraspinal structures, such as the vertebrae, muscles, perineum, and skin (103). Finally, a third hypothesis assumes that ectopic ependymomas derive from "heterotopic" ependymal cell remnants located within the sacral region (1). A further point in favor of a dysembryoblastic process is the frequent association of these tumors with *spina bifida*.

There is a bimodal age distribution with the first peak occurring under 8 years of age and the second in the fourth decade (85). Clinical manifestations depend on localization of the tumors. Ependymomas situated posteriorly to the sacrum usually present with a local mass, whereas those situated in the pelvis almost invariably induce bowel and bladder dysfunction. Local pain or pain with a sciatic nerve distribution is also a relatively frequent complaint.

Plain x-ray and conventional tomographic examinations usually reveal some degree of sacral erosion. Computed tomography scanning with intrathecal administration of contrast medium and CSF protein examination helps to differentiate ectopic ependymomas from the more common intradural ependymomas of the conus medullaris-cauda equina region. A careful pelvic examination and a barium-enema cystoscopy or proctoscopy are also necessary. Complete excision of this type of tumor can occasionally be achieved in cases of ependymomas situated posteriorly to the sacrum. An anterior approach (or a combined anterior and posterior approach in cases of sacral erosion) is required for patients in whom ectopic ependymomas develop in the presacral or pelvic areas. Macroscopically, the tumors appear as well defined and often lobulated masses; histologically, they are of the papillary or myxopapillary type, although the presence of more anaplastic cells can be demonstrated in some cases (85). Local recurrence is common and systemic metastases have been reported as well (78,103).

Dysplastic spinal tumors associated with Recklinghausen's disease are rare in children, except in cases of generalized neurofibromatosis. When the spinal roots are involved, the tumors can develop within the spinal canal, often assuming a dumbbell configuration. Malignant degeneration in the pediatric age is uncommon. It is worth pointing out, however, that in children with Recklinghausen's disease, associated mesodermal defects may produce x-ray changes of the spine similar to those induced by the presence of a tumor, such as a scalloping of the vertebral bodies, enlargement of intervertebral foramina, or the protrusion of a dilated dural sac or root sleeves (dural ectasia) mimicking dumbbell tumors (48).

Tumors Related to Peripheral Nerves, Roots, and Meninges

Although these tumors represent the most common form (50% to 60%) of intraspinal tumors in adults, they are relatively rare in children, in whom they account for about 15% of cases (64,71). Two thirds of them are neurilemmomas and neurofibromas, and the remainder are meningiomas and the rare ependymomas of the cauda equina and filum terminale.

Neurilemmomas and Neurofibromas

These neoplasms arise from the dorsal roots at all spinal levels with segmental, multisegmental, multicentric (neurofibromatosis), and hourglass features (107). Neurinomas, due to the proliferation of Schwann cells in the form of an isolated tumor, occur typically in older children; they are exceptional in infants. As in adults, there is a slight preponderance in the thoracic region and in the lateroposterior aspect of the spinal canal. These tumors are more often confined exclusively within the intradural space (76%) and less frequently assume an intradural-extradural hourglass configuration (23%). Only in a few instances (less than 1%) do they develop completely within the extradural space (64). Giant neurinomas extending over two or more vertebral segments are slightly more frequent in the pediatric population (14%) than in adults (10%).

The most common presenting complaint is radicular pain, which in this age group is characteristically associated with spinal stiffness or deviation of the vertebral column. Contrary to what occurs in adults, the clinical evolution in children is relatively rapid. In almost half the cases plain X-ray examinations of the spine reveal the thinning of the vertebral pedicles and scalloping of the posterior vertebral bodies (Fig. 3.4). In no case, however, does the erosion proceed to the complete destruction of the osseous structures.

Bone abnormalities may be severe with an intradural tumor; they are less so in cases of hourglass neurinomas because of the more severe and progressive clinical manifestations of this type of lesion. Hourglass neurinomas are characteristically revealed by the enlargement of the intervertebral foramina (Figs. 3.5, 3.20A). Scoliosis or kyphoscoliosis is a commonly associated finding in this type of tumor, constituting the only clinical manifestation in about 20% of cases.

The basic neuroradiologic findings are very similar in both neurinomas and neurofibromas and neurofibrosarcomas (also called neurilsarcomas). Although myelography clearly depicts intradural lesions (Fig. 3.21) and the effect of extradural lesions on the dural sac and medulla, CT appears the method of choice for the demonstration of both intraspinal and ex-

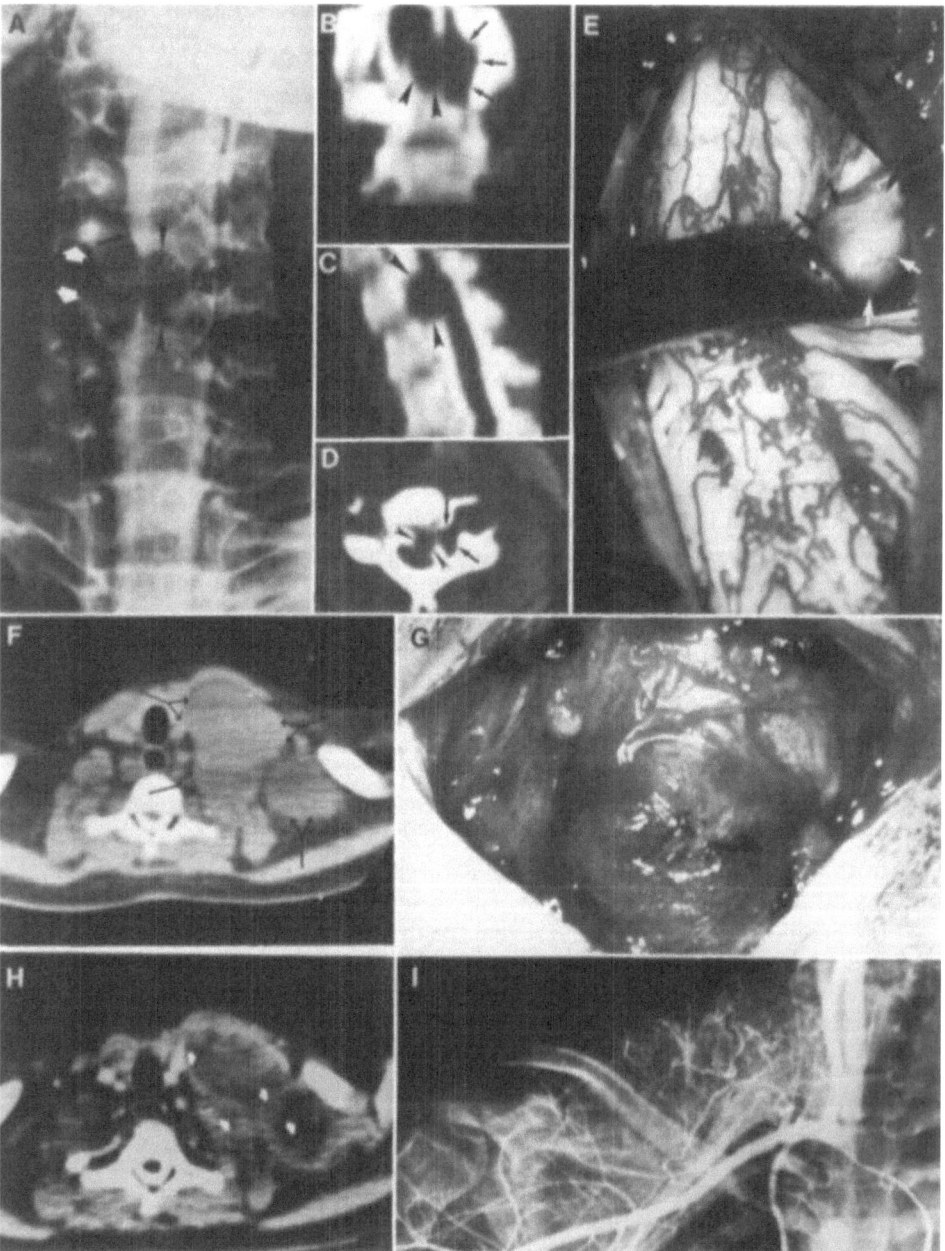

Figure 3.20. Hourglass malignant neurofibroma in an 11-year-old girl presenting with rapidly growing mass in the region of the right brachial plexus. **A** Cervical myelography reveals at C-4 to C-5 both a round extradural mass (*arrowheads*) and an extradural component (*arrows*) to right. Note that the right C-4 to C-5 neuroforamen is enlarged (*white arrows*). **B–D** Myelo-CT with coronal (**B**) and sagittal reformated images clearly define the relationships between the intradural

traspinal components. In particular, myelo-CT adds the advantages of myelography and CT, and intravenous (IV) enhancement further improves the visualization of extraspinal component (Figs. 3.5, 3.20). Generally speaking, most neurinomas and neurofibromas exhibit contrast enhancement after IV administration of the contrast medium (6,7,29); relatively hypodense areas within the tumor (necrosis) are encountered in both benign and malignant tumors when they reach a large size, and this criterion cannot be used in the differential diagnosis. However, in malignant neurilsarcomas, necrotic and pseudocystic areas are very frequent and correspond to the angiographic picture of malignant vascularization (Fig. 3.20).

In patients with Recklinghausen's neurofibromatosis and enlarged foramina or scalloped vertebral bodies, CT is essential to differentiate dural ectasias (and meningoceles) from hourglass or intradural neurofibromas (Fig. 3.22). The neuroradiological finding of multiple neurofibromas is also specific for Recklinghausen's disease when there is no clear evidence of cutaneous lesions. In most of these patients surgical excision of intradural, extradural, and extraspinal lesions is followed by recurrence.

Although there has been limited experience in MRI diagnosis of spinal neurinomas/neurofibromas, the MRI findings of these tumors are the same as for intracranial areas: the neurinomas appear hyperintense in T1-weighted images in comparison with the CSF-containing thecal sac (Fig. 3.4), and the use of paramagnetic agents [gadolinium, diethylenetriamine pentaacetic acid (DTPA)] greatly enhances their MR intensity and demonstration. It is very important to stress the need of multiplane images because the use of the one sagittal MRI view may result in an erroneous diagnosis of intramedullary tumor (39,99) (Fig. 3.22). Spinal taps may also contribute significantly to the diagnosis by revealing the characteristic

◁————————————————————————————————————

component (*arrowheads*), and the extradural component (*arrows*) of the tumor and the displaced cord. In the axial slices the tumor extends within the spinal canal via the enlarged neuroforamen. E In this surgical view the intradural part of the tumor is well visualized (*arrows*). The intraspinal component of the tumor could be completely excised. Histology revealed "highly cellular" neurofibroma. F Axial slice at the level of the brachial plexus region demonstrates the huge extraspinal lobulated mass (*arrows*). G Corresponding surgical view shows the surface of the tumor. The lesion was subsequently removed by microsurgical technique without neurologic deficit and with minimal residual tumor. H,I After one year the patient presents with an obvious recurrence of the supraclavicular mass and CT confirms the explosive recurrence with large hypodense areas of necrosis (*white arrows* in H). Angiography demonstrates the typical malignant vascularization and the adhesion of the tumor to the brachiocephalic vessels. Despite repeated surgical approaches, chemotherapy, and radiotherapy, the patient subsequently died.

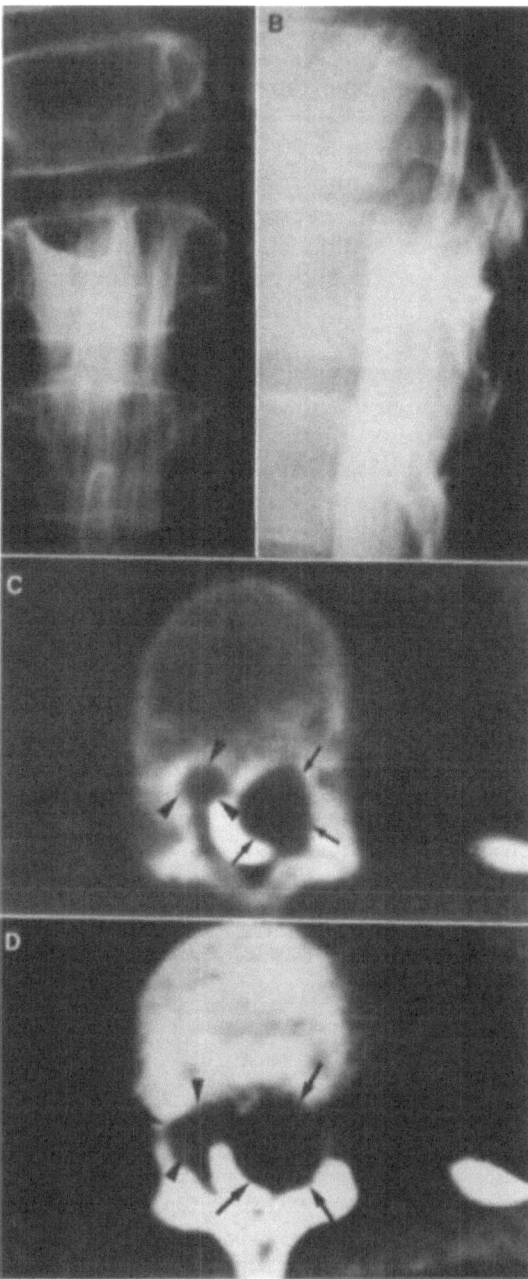

Figure 3.21. Purely intradural neurinoma at L-1 (8-year-old boy). **A,B** Myelography discloses complete block at L-1 resulting from an intradural mass. **C,D** Myelo-CT better outlines the extramedullary tumor (*arrows*) and the displaced cord (*arrowheads*).

increase in protein content. Cerebrospinal fluid proteins may, in fact, reach values as high as 10 g/ml or more.

Total excision of the tumor is necessary to prevent recurrence; separate operative approaches may be needed for the intraspinal and extraspinal components, especially at the cervical level. Neurilemmomas and neurinomas are relatively avascular, ovoid masses that usually are intimately related with a dorsal root; a section of this structure is thus required after clipping it above and below the tumor itself. The operation may be difficult in cases of giant neurinomas of the cauda equina, which often develop from many sensory and motor roots. Ten percent of the intraspinal neurinomas in all ages are part of a generalized neurofibromatosis. In the pediatric population, however, a higher proportion than that reported above is found (64). The intraspinal neurinomas developing in young patients with Recklinghausen's disease are typically found in older children, assume an hourglass configuration, and are distributed along the spinal axis with a slight preference for the cervical region. Though cases of Recklinghausen's disease have been reported without the cutaneous stigmata, the skin anomalies (café au lait spots, subcutaneous noduli, molluscum pendulum) usually facilitate the diagnosis in patients complaining of radicular pain and spinal stiffness, as well as presenting with a deviation of the spine. The differential diagnosis includes other tumors that may be associated with a blastomatosis, such as meningiomas, ganglioneuromas, and lipomas. While a complete surgical excision of the isolated neurinomas is often obtained, significant difficulties are usually faced in cases of multiple neurinomas, which may require several different approaches, or in patients with diffuse neurofibromatosis.

Meningiomas

These tumors are rare in infancy and childhood, accounting for only 3% to 4% of all intraspinal tumors in contrast with 25% as reported in adults (25,26,49). In children these tumors exhibit an obvious preference for the 10- to 15-year-age group (64) and show some differences when compared with adults, namely, the absence of the clear predominance for females and for the thoracic region, the relatively low incidence of the "psammomatous" type, and the less frequent association with neurofibromatosis. Multiple meningiomas are exceptional in the pediatric population, both in children with and without Recklinghausen's disease (26,85,96). Multicentric neoplastic foci, the spreading of neoplastic cells along CSF pathways, and the diffusion of the tumor by venous routes have been proposed as possible pathogenic mechanisms accounting for the occurrence of these tumors at different spinal levels, as well as in intraspinal and intracranial compartments in the same patient (96,103).

Although the time interval (18 months) between the onset of symptoms and diagnosis is considerably shorter in children than in adults, clinical manifestations of intraspinal meningiomas in this age group may long re-

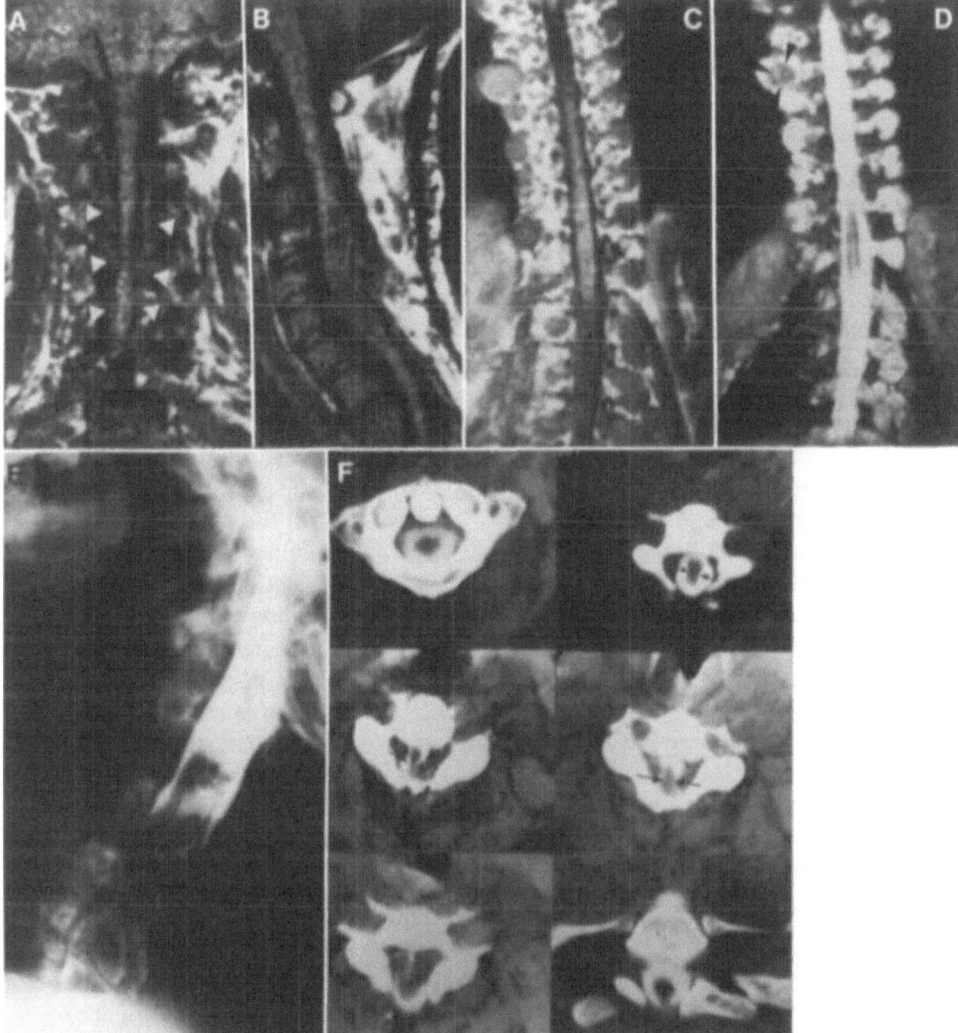

Figure 3.22. Multiple recurrent neurofibromas of the cervical spine in a 16-year-old boy with Recklinghausen's disease and multiple lateral thoracic meningoceles. Previous excision of cervical neurofibromas was performed 7 years prior to the examination. **A,B** Coronal and sagittal T1-weighted MRIs of the cervical spine. There is a decrease of the coronal (**A**) diameter of the spinal cord, which, by turns, shows an increased sagittal (**B**) diameter. In **A** isohypointense areas contour the middle cervical cord (*arrowheads*). **C,D** Coronal T1-(**C**) and T2 (**D**)-weighted images of the same patient disclose multiple outpouchings of the subarachnoid space through the neuroforamina. Note that all the outpouchings (representing lateral meningoceles) have the same signal of the CSF in both T-1 and T-2 images; only in the largest right meningocele there is an area of relative hypointensity (*arrowheads*) in the T2-weighted image; this finding suggests the presence of a vegetating neurofibroma within the meningocele. **E** Laterocervical myelography in the lateral

main subtle or assume a puzzling character. Painful spinal rigidity is the most common clinical complaint. In some patients, however, only walk fatigability over a period of several months is reported (26,64,78).

Pediatric spinal meningiomas do not show any typical findings, and in general they look like the more common neurinomas (Fig. 3.23). However, calcifications are more frequently encountered in meningiomas, and sometimes one can observe an area of sclerosis in the bony attachment of the tumor. In most cases plain X-ray study demonstrates only the non-specific finding of an intraspinal mass lesion. Myelo-CT once again appears to be the most complete method. Further, meningiomas display positive contrast enhancement (6,29,72) whereas intracranial and intraspinal meningiomas exhibit the same MRI intensity of the nervous parenchyma; this finding limits the usefulness of MRI in the diagnosis of meningiomas (80,99).

Complete surgical excision of the tumor is the keystone in the treatment. The operation is more difficult in those cases where the meningioma has developed anteriorly to the spinal cord than in those where the tumor is situated laterally or ventrolaterally. The excision "en masse" of anterior meningiomas is, in fact, never possible, and a piecemeal intracapsular removal may be required (64). To prevent recurrences, the implantation area on the dura and on the nerve root eventually engulfed in the tumor should also be removed.

Ependymomas of the Filum Terminale

These tumors, probably arising from the ependyma of the central canal, may be discrete and so mobile in some instances as to simulate a neurofibroma. In such cases the ependymoma assumes a globoid configuration that makes it barely distinguishable from a neurofibroma attached to a nerve root of the cauda equina. In other cases the tumors are spindle-shaped and extend for several vertebral metameres (Figs. 3.24-3.26) along the middle of the nerve roots. The "en bloc" removal of this type of ependymoma is almost always possible, and dissection must be started very cautiously from the upper pole of the tumor to avoid traction on the conus medullaris; care must be taken to protect the nerve roots with cotton pledgets soaked in physiological saline (48). Nevertheless, because of the considerable space available for their growth, ependymomas developing

◁————————————————————————————————

projection resembles the sagittal MRI (B) with apparent widening of the cord. F Myelo-CT (axial slices from C-1 to T-1) well outlines the pathological anatomy of the cervical area: from C-3 to C-7 multiple neurofibromatous masses are demonstrated flattening the cord (*arrows*) from both sides and reducing its coronal diameter. The masses are predominantly extradural, and the dural sac protrudes posteriorly through the laminectomy.

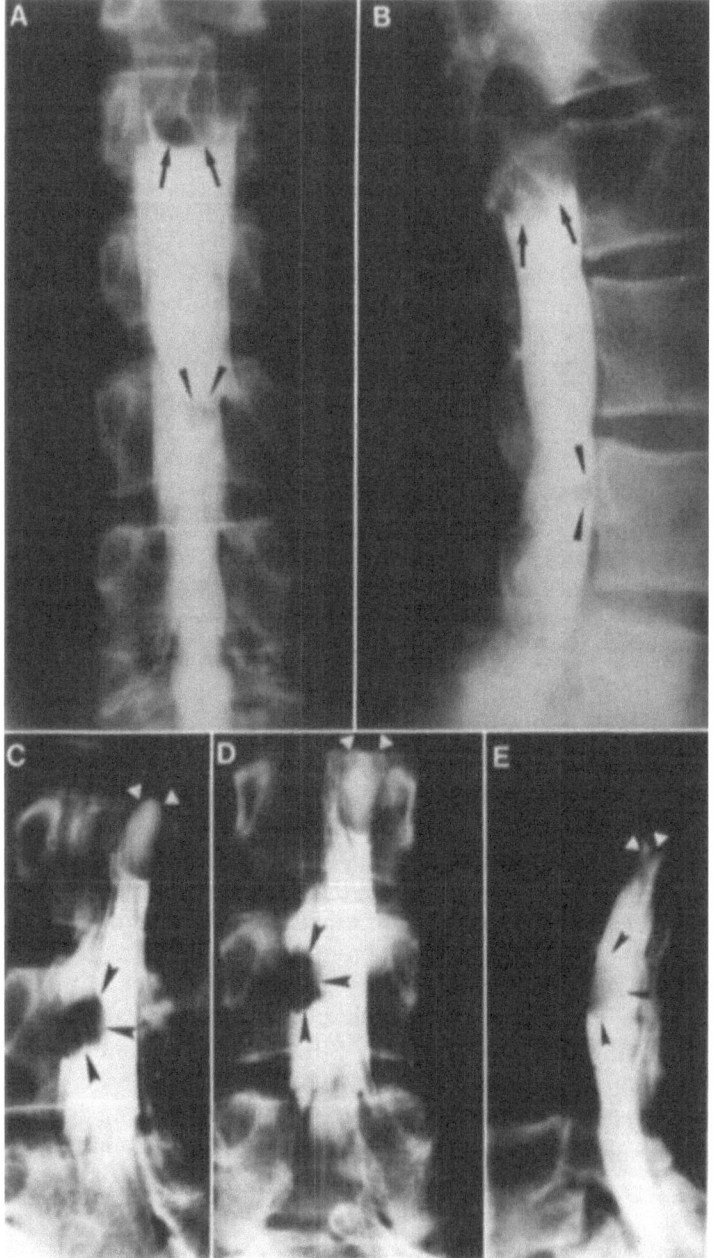

Figure 3.23. Multiple spinal meningiomas. This patient had been operated on because of intradural spinal meningioma at L-4 when 8 years old. After 4 years of complete clinical recovery, she again experienced lumbar and radicular pain and leg weakness. Repeat myelography (**A,B**) demonstrated a new intradural mass at L-2 level, inducing a complete CSF block (*arrows*). The site of the previous op-

at the cauda equina level may remain clinically silent and eventually increase to a giant size. A spinal tap revealing the considerably increased protein content in the CSF and the radiological changes simulating those of giant neurinomas may significantly contribute to the diagnosis even when the clinical symptoms are mild. The total removal of this latter type of tumor, although difficult because of its hemorrhagic nature (Fig. 3.24C), is mandatory in order to prevent recurrence. Careful microsurgical dissection, under magnification, of each single nerve root from the tumoral tissue is absolutely necessary.

Extrinsic Malignant Tumors

This heterogeneous group of tumors constitutes 10% to 20% of all myeloradicular compressions in children. With the exception of neuroblastomas, there are three types of sarcomas: reticulosarcoma, sarcoma X, and lymphosarcoma, which account for more than two thirds of the cases of extrinsic malignant tumors, followed by metastases and hemolymphopathies (18). These figures differ significantly from those in adults, where metastatic lesions make up the large majority of spinal epidural tumors.

Sarcomas

Sarcomas are rare in infants under 1 year of age, but become more common in children aged from 10 to 15 years, with a small predominance in females. They are derived from soft tissues as well as from the adjacent chondral and bone structures. In several instances, however, the histological identification is impossible to establish (15). These tumors usually extend over several vertebral levels, with an apparent major incidence in the cervical and upper thoracic regions. The most common presenting complaints are spinal and radicular pain in more than half the patients and sensory and motor deficits in about a sixth of the patients. In other instances, the tumor is accidentally discovered in children during the investigation of unexplained fever or spine injury. The course of symptoms is usually progressive, although an abrupt worsening may be recorded in some patients.

<hr/>

eration was marked by a small filling defect at L-4 (*arrowheads*). A second operation was carried out with excision of another intradural meningioma and good clinical result. Three years after the last operation, the patient presented with recurrence of her symptoms. A new myelogram was performed (**C,D,E**) showing an extradural block at L-2 to L-3 level (*white arrowheads*) as well as a more caudal filling defect (*black arrowheads*). At surgery all the abnormalities appeared related to an adhesive arachnoiditis.

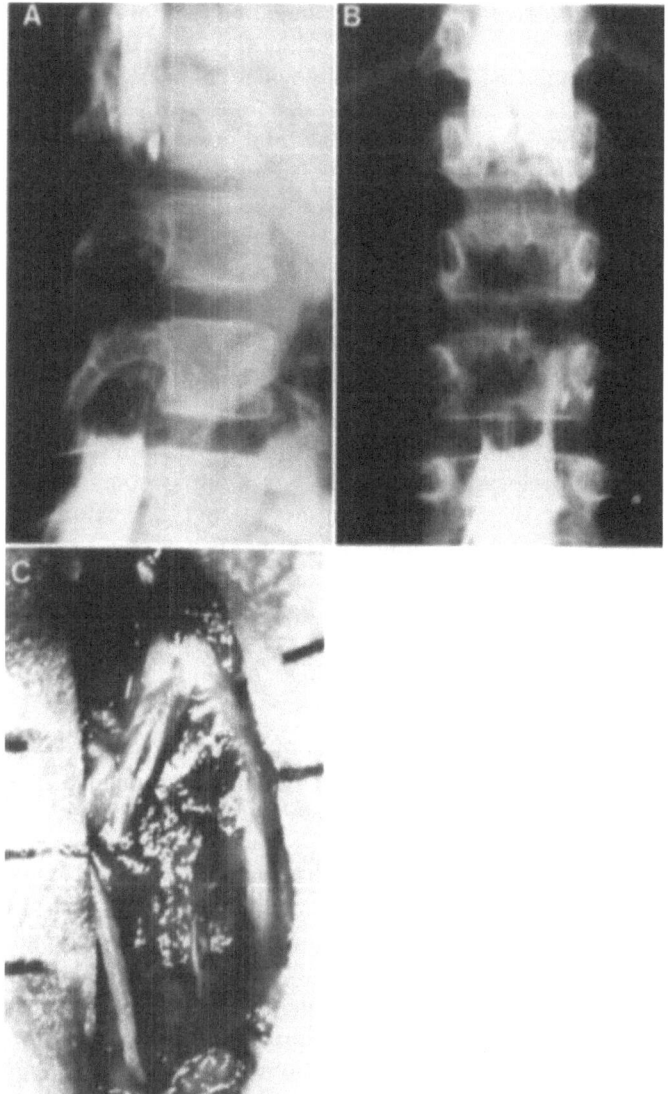

Figure 3.24. Ependymoma of the filum terminale in a 7-year-old girl **A,B** Myelography. A double introduction of the contrast medium was necessary, above
and below the lesion, in order to demonstrate both upper and lower pole of the
intradural tumor extending from L-1 to L-4. **C** At surgery the tumor appears extensively hemorrhagic.

Figure 3.25. Ependymoma of the filum terminale. **A,B** Myelographic evidence of ▷
an intradural mass with its upper pole at L-2. **C,D** Multiecho SE sequence allows
only a poor distinction of the tumor, which exhibits the same intensity of the CSF.
A good demonstration of the tumor could probably be obtained by means of proper
surface coil.

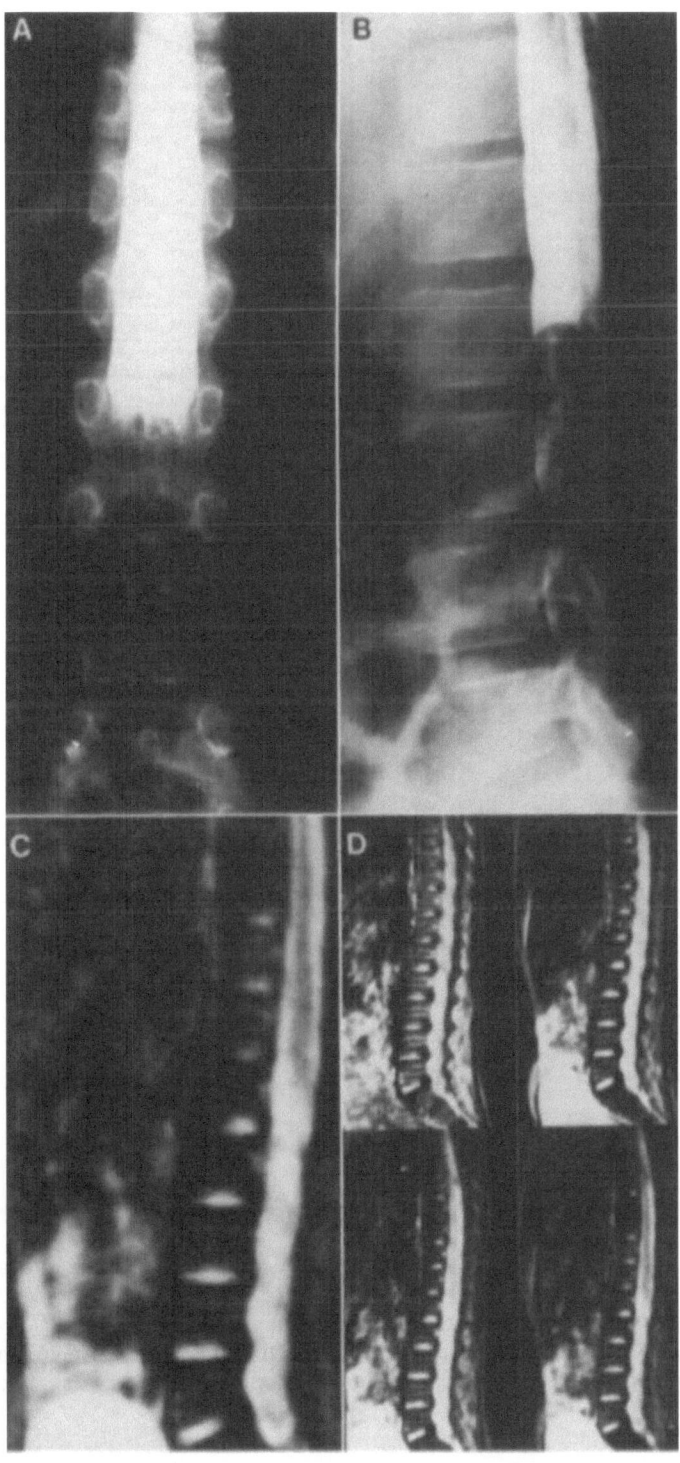

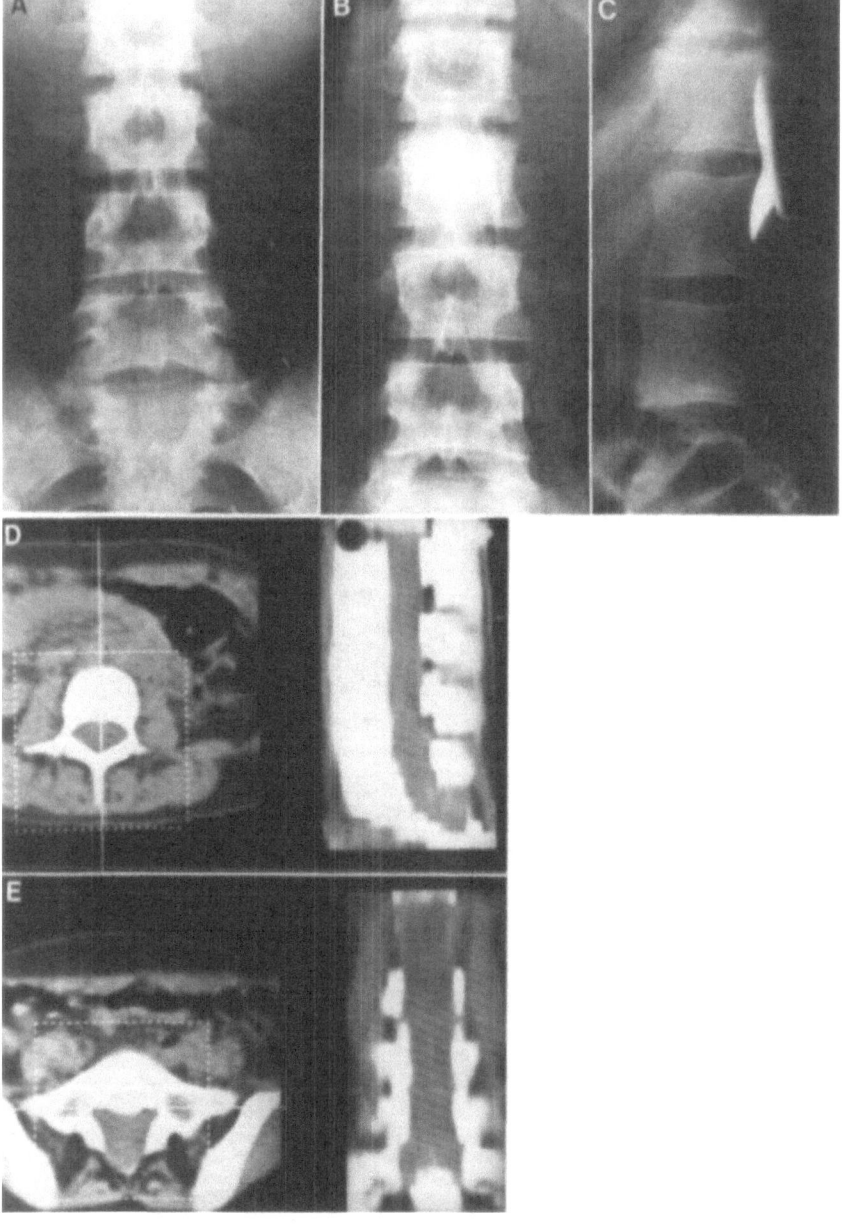

Figure 3.26. Ependymoma of the filum terminale. **A** AP view of the lumbar spine demonstrates marked thinning of the pedicles of L-3 and L-2. **B,C** At myelography there is a complete block at L-2 resulting from an intradural mass. **D,E** Myelo-CT with sagittal and coronal reformation fails to detect contrast medium below the myelographic block. At surgery an intradural ependymoma was found extending from L-2 to S-1.

In about a fourth of these children the appearance of a paravertebral in-
dolent subcutaneous mass can be noticed during the course of the disease.

At the radiological examination, half the patients exhibit areas of vertebral osteolysis but rarely of bone hyperdensity. The radiological anomalies, however, are nearly always confined to one vertebral body, despite the usually large extension of the tumor. Computed tomography and
myelography may define the exact extent of the lesion as well as the spinal
cord compression (Fig. 3.27). Treatment consists of decompressive laminectomy with excision of the tumoral mass as complete as possible, and
radiotherapy. A 5-year-survival is reached in less than a fifth of cases.

Metastatic Tumors

These tumors can be subdivided into two main groups: metastases from
the seeding of neoplastic cells through the cerebrospinal fluid and blood-
borne metastases. The recurrence of metastases from intracranial tumors
seeded along the CSF pathways is common in cases of medulloblastomas
(105). A 33% rate of metastases has been reported with this type of tumor,
almost all of them being intraspinal and only a few intracranial (70). Such
a high percentage of metastatic spinal lesions justifies the current practice
of administering radiotherapy to the whole spine in children operated on
because of medulloblastomas in the posterior cranial fossa.

The second most common intracranial tumors to seed are ependymomas,
with a rate of 31.6% of spinal metastases (109), and choroid plexus pap-
illomas, with a rate of 20% (56). They are followed by retinoblastomas
(17.6%), pineal neoplasms, astrocytomas, and lymphomas (13). The above-
mentioned rates are mainly based on autopsy observations, but with the
advent of water-soluble contrast myelography, they have been confirmed
in vivo especially when using nonionic contrast medium (23,30,105) in the
supine position (because of the prevalently dorsal location of this type of
lesion).

Myelographic findings (Figs. 3.28, 3.29) consist of nodularity and ir-
regularity of the distal sac and nerve roots, as well as obliteration of the
root sleeves in cases of lumbosacral metastases. On the other hand, in
the cervical and thoracic regions the anomalies mainly reflect the involvement of the cord, with its obvious widening (Fig. 3.30) (105). In some
children with widespread meningeal involvement, the myelographic picture
is similar to that of adhesive arachnoiditis.

Myelography can be completed by myelo-CT, especially when there is
a complete CSF block. Today, MRI easily reveals intramedullary metastases (Fig. 3.31) without hazard and so it is the time to propose the routine
use of MRI in all patients with medulloblastoma or ependymoma of the
posterior fossa to obtain a complete staging of the disease (87).

The pathogenetic hypotheses include ependymal breaching by the primary tumor, or associated hydrocephalus favoring the subarachnoid
seeding and fragmentation of the tumor bathed in CSF, eventually facil-

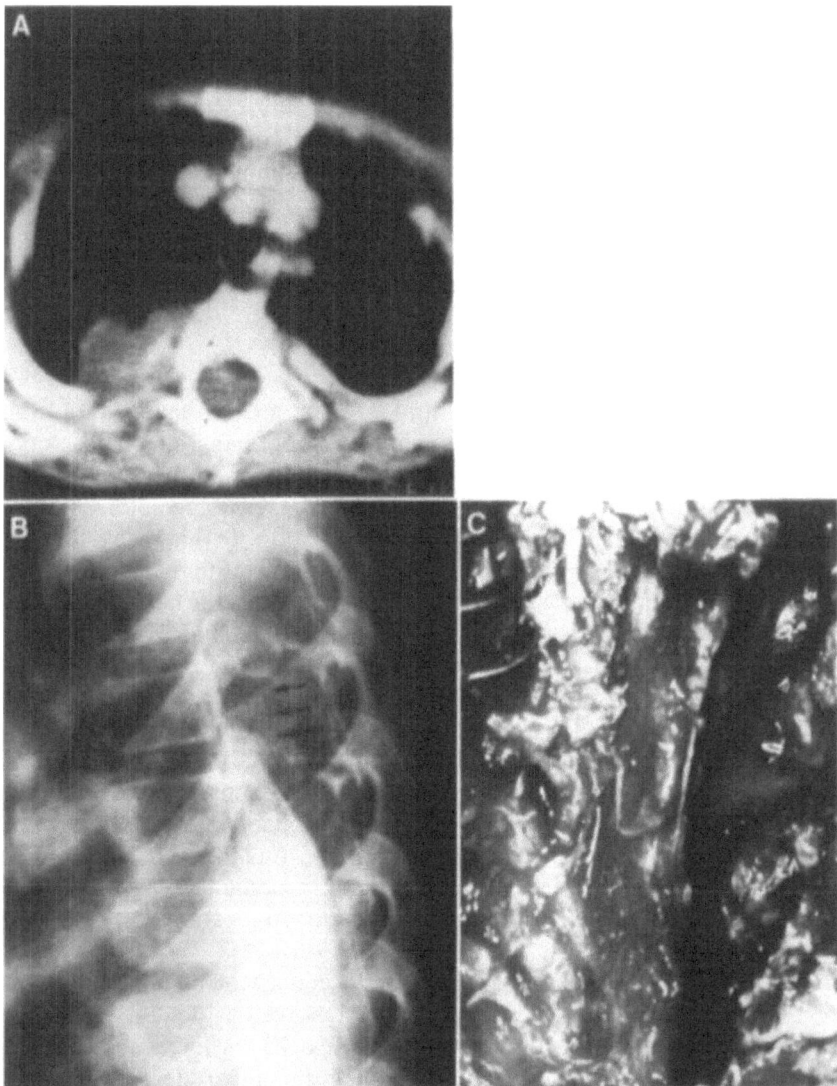

Figure 3.27. Indifferentiated sarcoma of the mediastinum in a 4-year-old boy. **A** Intravenous-enhanced CT shows the tumor infiltrating the right costovertebral joint and occupying the spinal canal. **B** Myelography shows a complete CSF block due to an extradural mass at D-5. Note destruction of the posterior vertebral elements (*arrows*). **C** Intraoperative view of the tumor.

itated by trauma or surgical manipulation (19,110). It is worth stressing, however, that spinal metastases have been detected in some children already at the time of the original craniotomy, suggesting that spreading may have already begun before the initial surgery.

Radiotherapy is still the main method of treatment, as surgical excision

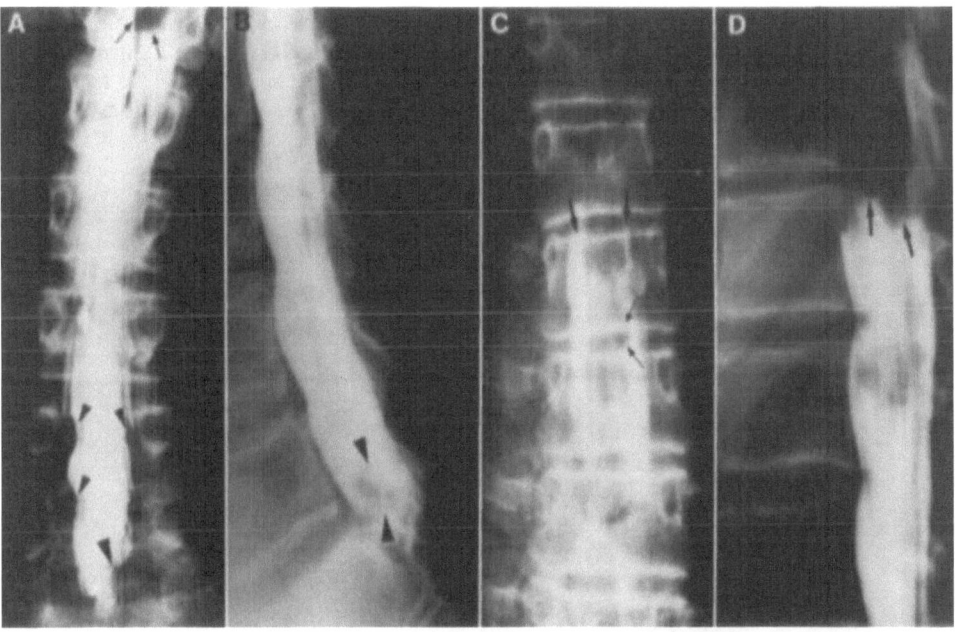

△ **Figure 3.28.** Diffuse spinal metastases from posterior
fossa medulloblastoma via CSF seeding. Myelography
demonstrates multiple seedings both in the lumbosacral area (*arrowheads* in **A,B**) and in the dorsal
region resulting in an uncomplete block at D-11,
complete block at D-8 (*large arrows* in **C,D**), and
irregularities of the cord surface (*small arrows*).

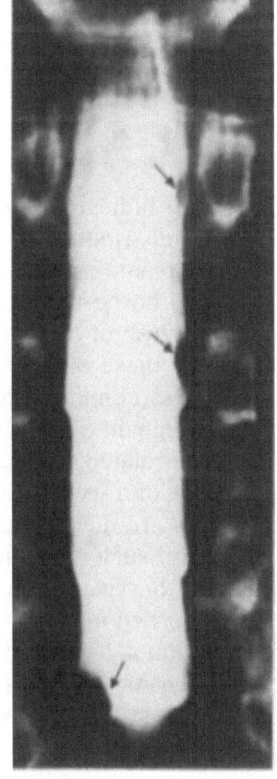

Figure 3.29. Multiple small metastatic deposits in the
cauda equina in 12-year-old boy with ventricular
ependymoblastoma. The metastases (*arrows*) appear
as small filling defects at the level of the merging
roots.

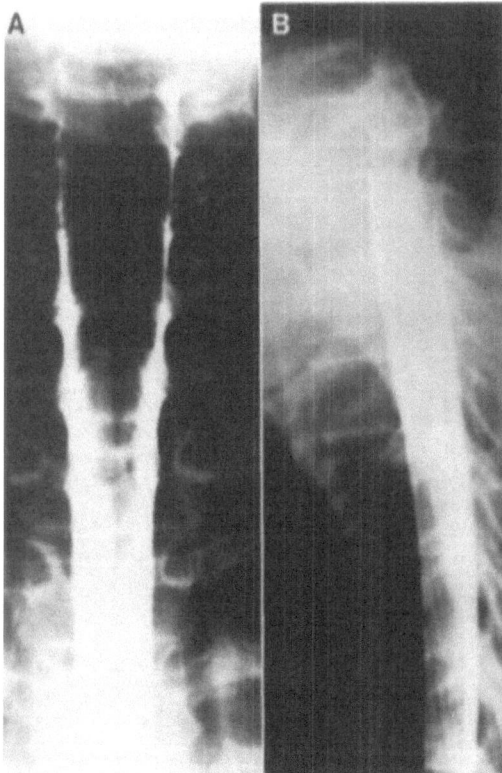

Figure 3.30. Myelographic demonstration of intrinsic cervical cord metastasis from vermian medulloblastoma.

is rarely indicated. In fact, spinal metastases, even when discrete, are usually distributed along the whole spinal axis and are intimately related to the spinal cord, which is often infiltrated as well.

Blood-borne metastases are considerably less frequent, varying from 10% to 20% of all extrinsic malignant compressive lesions of the spine. Most of these originate from bone sarcomas, especially of the reticular type; less common are the metastatic localizations of nephroblastomas and malignant ovarian teratomas. Girls are more affected than boys, with two age-related peaks, respectively, from 1 to 5 and from 10 to 15 years of age. Contrary to other types of secondary malignant lesions, these metastases are never associated with clinical manifestations but give signs abruptly, such as a sudden paraplegia, during the course of the primary disease. Survival, even in patients operated on, is very short: 75% of deaths are recorded in the first 6 postoperative months, and all patients usually die within a 2-year period. Radiotherapy has a merely palliative role.

Malignant meningitis, especially in infants with lymphoblastic leukemia, is the most common form of spinal involvement in cases of hemolymphopathies. However, in adolescents with acute myeloblastic leukemia it is not unusual to find invasion of the epidural space in the form of multifocal masses that compress the spinal cord (113). In almost all of these patients the neurological manifestations, which are similar to those of epidural sarcomas, constitute the revealing clinical signs of the condition. Results of the management of these lesions, whether surgical or radio- and chemotherapeutic, are deceiving, with almost all patients dying within 18 months, irrespective of the treatment performed. Conversely, the results that can be obtained in the rare cases of spinal metastatic lesions due to Hodgkin's disease are more satisfactory and are considerably more responsive to radiation therapy. In these latter cases, however, surgical decompressive procedures should be limited in patients who present with a rapidly progressive paralysis.

Tumors originating from the autonomic nervous system (sympathetic ganglia, adrenal gland) may enter the spinal canal through the intervertebral foramina, assuming a dumbbell configuration. In infants, the extraspinal component may reach very large proportions, and it characteristically develops posteriorly to the spine in the posterolateral pharyngeal region, within the mediastinal and retroperitoneal space. At the most caudal level, however, these tumors may occupy the presacral region. Usually, the tumor penetrates through several intervertebral foramina, reaching the epidural space, extending over several levels, and displacing the dural sac contralaterally (61). More rarely, the tumor envelopes and compresses all around the dural sac. Although the spinal dura is never infiltrated, roots and related vessels at the intervertebral foramen are intimately engulfed by the neoplastic tissue. Signs of spinal cord compression dominate the clinical picture: the paraplegia, often associated with pain, is usually rapidly progressive; it may be preceded in infants by an obvious stiffness of the spine or scoliosis.

Plain X-ray films may demonstrate the possible enlargement of the foramina and the soft-tissue mass in the paravertebral region; in some cases of malignant metastatic neuroblastoma, true metastases result in bone vertebral osteolysis. Nevertheless, myelo-CT appears mandatory when a patient presents with signs of medullary compression (2), for it allows the demonstration of the intraspinal (usually extradural) involvement as well as the extraspinal component (Fig. 3.32). Myelo-CT may be replaced by MRI when available (102).

Of the three main oncotypes that characterize this type of tumor, the neuroblastoma and ganglioneuroblastoma are highly malignant and are infiltrating when they occur in older children. Conversely, in a significant proportion of infants they show a favorable evolution, and spontaneous stabilization or complete regression can be observed in 10% of cases. Outcomes are improved with a complete excision of the pathologic tissue, followed by radiation and chemotherapy.

The third type of tumor, the ganglioneuroma (Fig. 3.6), represents the mature form, thus differing considerably from neuroblastomas and gan-

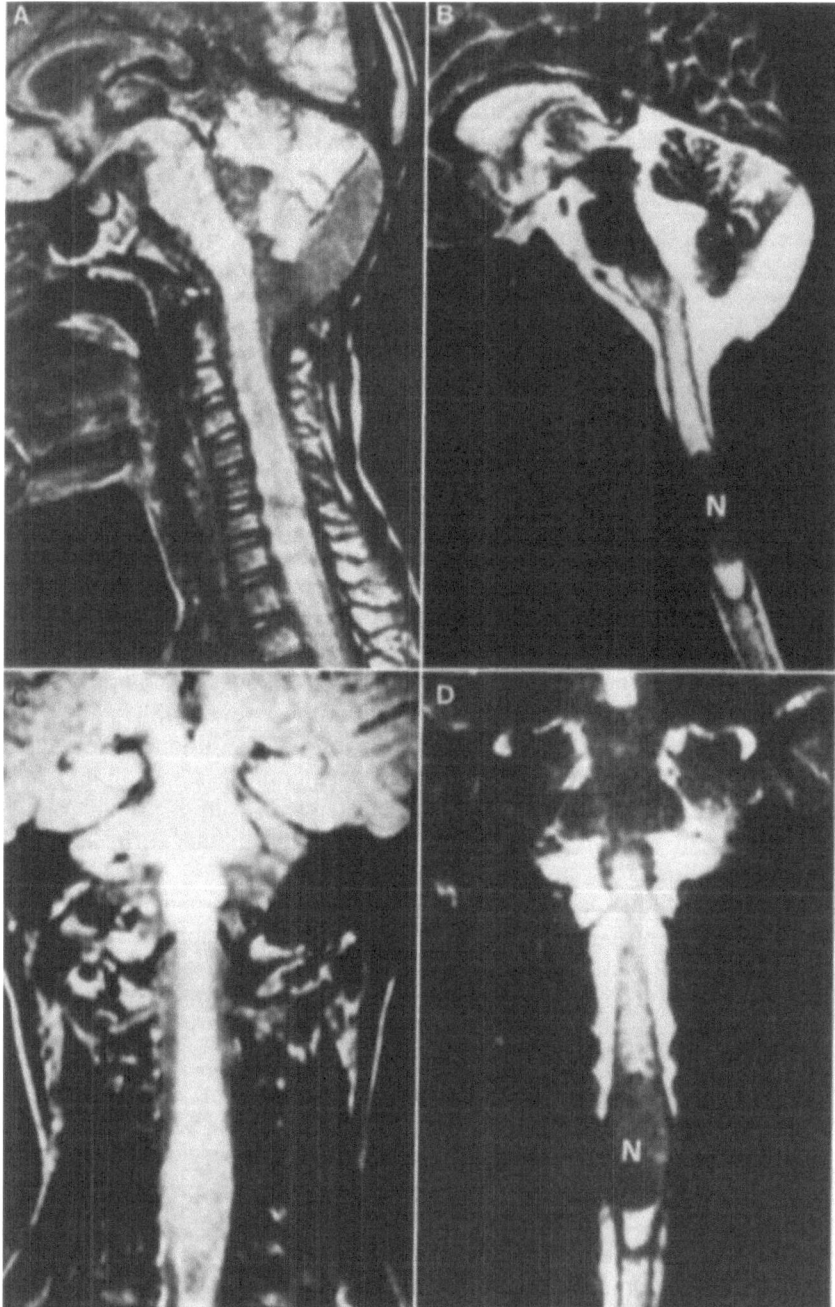

Figure 3.31. Medulloblastoma of the cerebellar vermis metastatizing to the cervical cord. This 10-year-old boy was operated on with complete excision of the medulloblastoma; despite radiotherapeutic prophylaxis 6 months after surgery the patient complained of progressive tetraparesis. **A,B** T1 and T2-weighted sagittal MRIs

glioneuroblastomas in prognosis. Ganglioneuromas are, in fact, benign and surgically treatable. They characteristically occur in older children, develop in a dumbbell configuration, and may be completely removed and cured with staged intraspinal and extraspinal approaches.

Vertebral Tumors

Tumors of the vertebrae are a relatively rare cause of spinal cord compression in children. The benign varieties include aneurysmal bone cysts, osteomas, chondromas, vertebral angiomas, and eosinophilic granulomas. Osteogenic sarcomas represent the malignant variety, together with the less common Ewing's sarcomas.

Aneurysmal Bone Cysts

These are essentially characterized by an expanding cystic lesion formed of an "extravertebral," firm reddish tissue, limited by a peripheral capsule. They should be regarded as a vascular malformation rather than a true neoplasm. Indeed, this type of lesion has been thought to depend on a local hemodynamic disturbance owing to an increase in venous pressure secondary to thrombosis, or else has been identified with a form of arteriovenous aneurysm or bone angioma. Other hypotheses regard aneurysmal bone cysts as a variety of myeloplaxis tumor, or as a reactive tissue developing after a trauma or in the presence of other bone anomalies (fibrocystic dysplasia, chondromyxoid fibromas). About half the cases are recorded in children and adolescents. The cervical and the lumbar regions of the spine are common locations (69). However, clinical manifestations more frequently characterize patients with thoracic lesions. Pain confined to the vertebrae, and limitations in the movement of the spine, often associated with torticollis, usually precede the neurological signs. Radicular pain is frequent in the lumbosacral localizations. Paraparesis is usually progressive, although a sudden appearance of paraplegia has been observed in some cases. The standard X-ray examination and tomography reveal the characteristic aspect of these tumors, which appears as a localized expansion of the bone that is formed by areas of central osteolysis, surrounded by thin, calcified cortical rims resembling an eggshell. The central osteolytic area may eventually be crossed by thin, irregularly calcified septa (Fig. 3.33).

◁

show expansion of the whole cervical cord with slight hypointensity in T-1 (**A**) while T-2 image outlines a central midcervical ovoid nodule (**N**) with the same hypointensity of the normal nervous tissue. More cranially and, to a lesser extent, more caudally there is a CSF-like hyperintensity that may represent edema, neoplastic infiltration, or cyst formation. **C,D** Coronal T1 and T2-weighted MRIs confirm the same signal behavior with central nodule (**N**) and global spindle like shape.

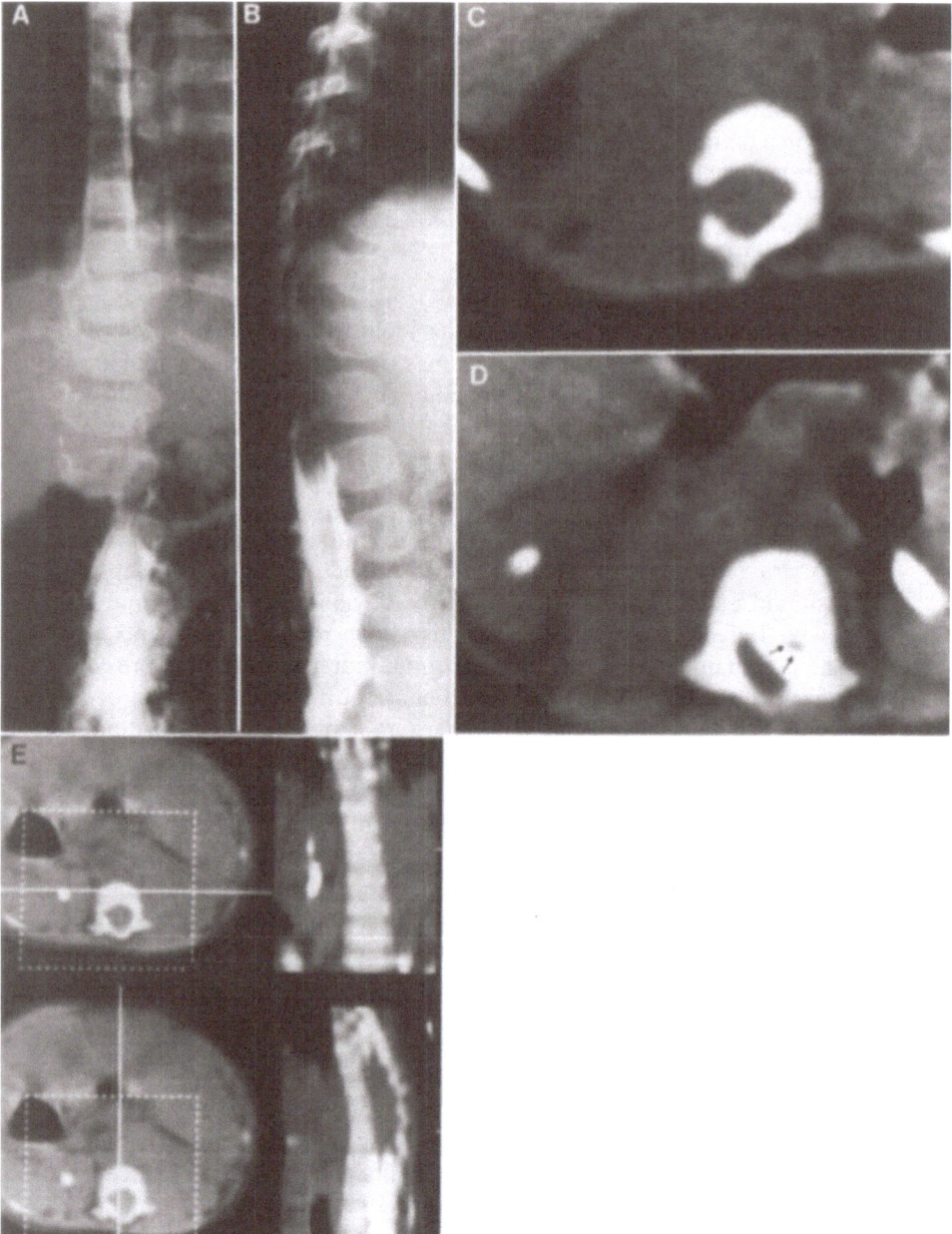

Figure 3.32. Paraspinal and intraspinal neuroblastoma in a 9-month-old child with rapidly progressive paraparesis. **A,B** Myelography demonstrates an extradural mass that completely occupies the spinal canal from L-2 to D-10. The dural sac is displaced contralaterally; the cord appears widened in **A** because of flattening. **C,D** Myelo-CT outlines a huge right paraspinal mass that extends in the spinal canal through the enlarged neuroforamen; the spinal canal in **A** is totally occupied by the tumor, and in **B** the cord is displaced toward left (*arrows*). Note that the right kidney is pushed laterally. **E** Coronal and sagittal reconstructions confirm the findings obtained by myelography and axial CT.

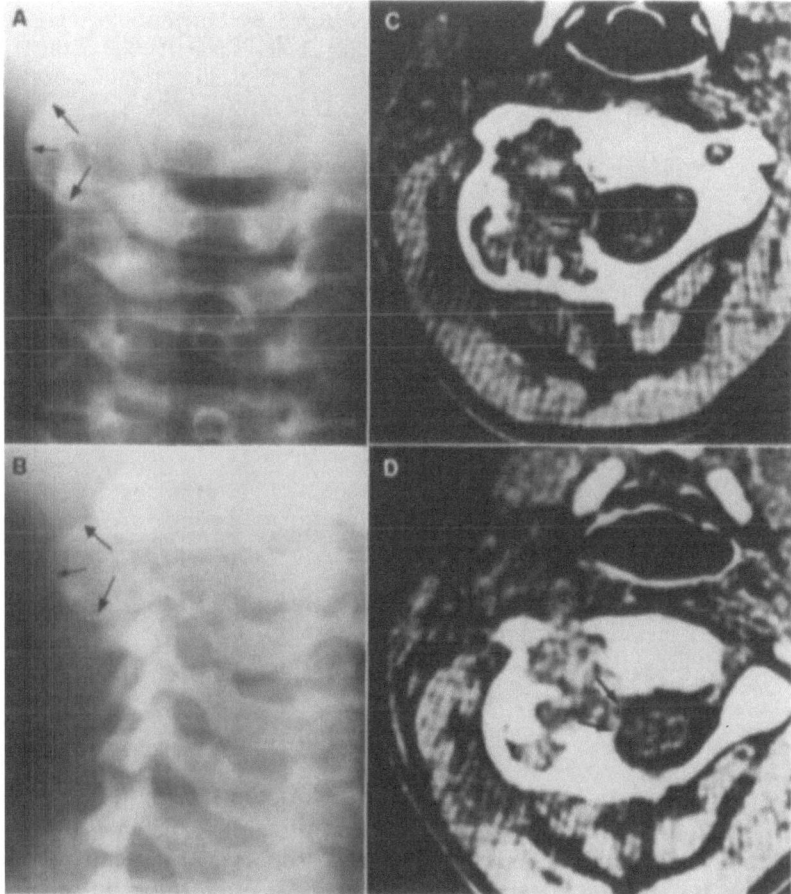

Figure 3.33. Aneurysmal bone cyst of C-2. **A,B** AP and oblique films of the cervical spine show an expansive lesion of the right transverse process and lamina (*arrows*). **C,D** Axial CT slices better define the expansion of the bone with sclerotic margins and enhancing hypervascular tissue. The inner bony contour of the spinal canal is disrupted (*arrows*), but the spinal cord is not yet compressed.

When the vertebral body is extensively involved, a pathological compression fracture may ensue (Fig. 3.34), resulting in spinal stenosis and spinal cord damage. The neural arch is most frequently involved, but the cysts developing at the level of the pedicles are those that more commonly induce cord compression. When untreated, aneurysmal bone cysts progressively invade all the vertebral segments and then extend to the adjacent superior and inferior vertebrae. Angiographic studies demonstrate a significant dilation of the afferent arterial branches associated with a

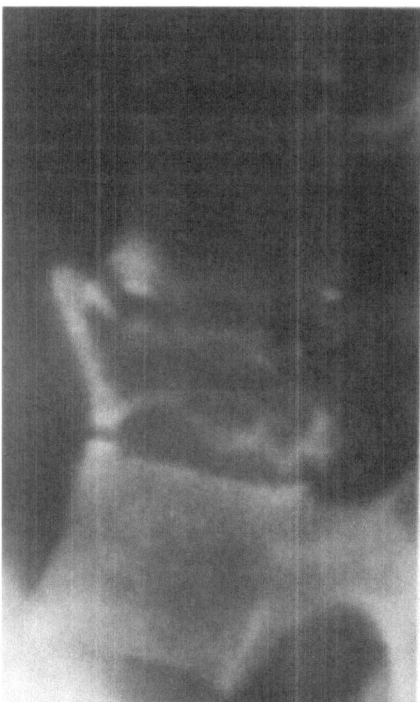

Figure 3.34. Lateral tomogram showing compression fracture of the D-10 vertebra resulting from aneurysmal cyst in a 12-year-old girl.

massive impregnation of the osseous lacuna. Although spontaneous healing of the lesion has been described, it is exceptionally rare, but abrupt deterioration of clinical conditions has been reported. Surgical treatment consists of removing the lesion (also curettage is often sufficient), relieving the compression of the nervous structure, and eventually stabilizing the spine. Radiotherapy has also proved to be effective, especially in cases where surgical treatment is difficult or appears insufficient. In fact, although recurrences are uncommon, they are not rare.

Also, *eosinophilic granulomas* of the spine (about 15% of the granulomas involving bones) are pseudotumoral benign lesions that may be part of a systemic process (histiocytosis X). When situated in the vertebrae (Fig. 3.35), eosinophilic granulomas are usually found in infants under 4 years of age, with no sex predominance; their clinical interest depends on the possible secondary compression of the adjacent nervous structures, as well as on the eventual alterations in the stability of the spine owing to the destruction of the vertebral bone. However, the occurrence of neurological signs is an extremely rare event. Furthermore, the lesion often evolves spontaneously from a stage of active proliferation of the eosinophilic cells to the healing stage, characterized by fibrotic reaction and bone regeneration. Consequently, a conservative attitude may be justified, especially in cases in which the lesion is confined to the posterior arch

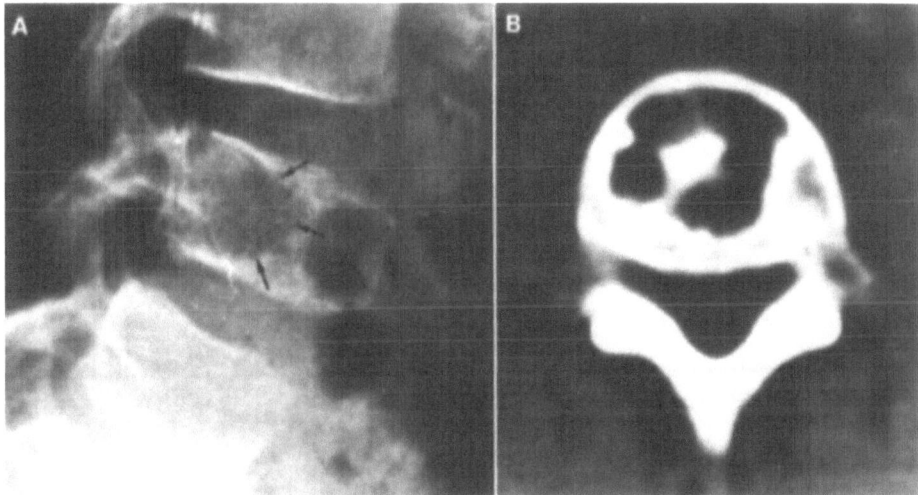

Figure 3.35. Eosinophilic granuloma of the L-4 vertebra. **A** Osteolytic area of the L-4 body with minimal decrease of the vertical diameter (*arrows*). **B** Unenhanced CT scan at the same level shows the "garlandlike" shape of the lesion.

of the vertebra. Curettage of the lesion or radiotherapy is also utilized with the aim of accelerating the reparative processes.

Osteomas, Chondromas, and Angiomas

These tumors are all very rare in the pediatric age. They typically occur in children aged 10 years or more and remain clinically silent for a long time. Thus, an accidental diagnosis is not rare after having carried out a radiological examination because of trauma. Nevertheless, associated scoliosis is frequent. Surgery is required only in cases of radicular or spinal cord compression. In asymptomatic patients, a wait-and-see policy is often adopted.

Bony malignant tumors affecting the spine are mainly osteogenic sarcomas (Fig. 3.36), Ewing's sarcomas (Fig. 3.37), and chondrosarcomas (Fig. 3.3). Standard X-ray films usually demonstrate only lytic and destructive changes, and the histological diagnosis is very difficult even by means of CT. The use of CT in these tumors results in a more complete evaluation of the intraspinal and extraspinal extension; again, myelo-CT is the method of choice and can further be improved by the combined use of IV contrast media. As in other extradural intraspinal lesions, it is obvious that myelo-CT is superior to conventional myelography in the definition of the intraspinal involvement (Figs. 3.36, 3.37). Moreover, CT is able to demonstrate minimal destructive vertebral changes in some areas (i.e., in the pelvis) in which conventional radiology has failed (Figs. 3.36, 3.37).

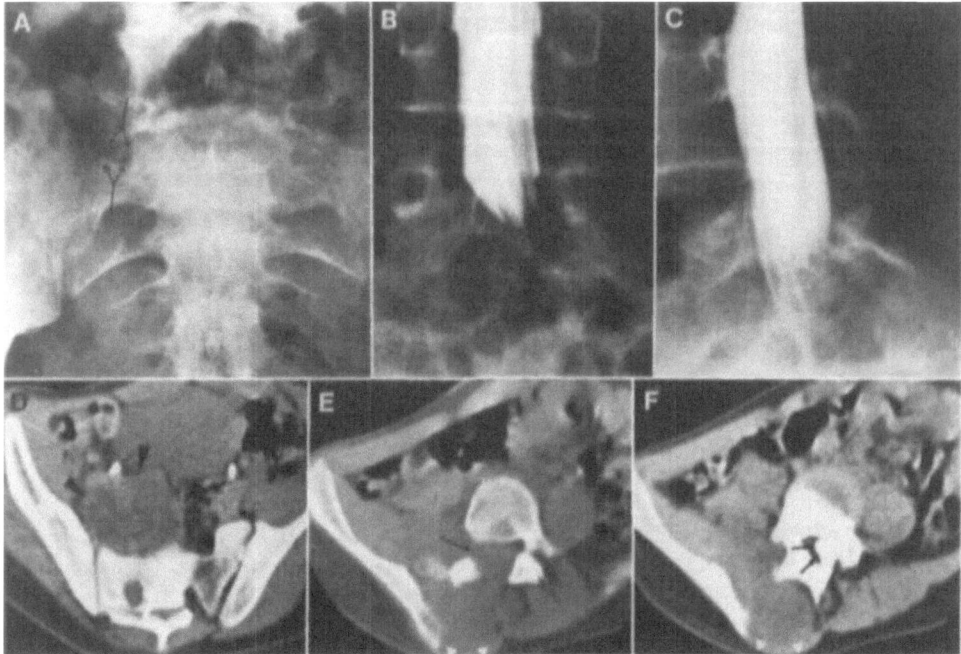

Figure 3.36. Twelve-year-old boy with S-1 radiculopathy and fever due to highly malignant osteogenic sarcoma of the sacrum. **A** Osteolysis in the right sacral wing (*arrows*) is difficult to detect. **B,C** Myelogram discloses a right extradural intraspinal mass with displacement of the dural sac. **D–F** Myelo-CT confirms the intraspinal involvement with displacement of the dural sac (*arrows* in **F**) and outlines a huge mass, with irregular enhancement, protruding in the pelvis from the eroded ventral surface of the right sacral wing (*arrowheads* in **D**); the ureter is displaced anteriorly. The tumor infiltrates the right iliac muscles as well as the posterior paraspinal muscle, resulting in a "bump" in the back (*white arrowheads* in **E** and **F**). At the L-5 level the tumor occupies completely the spinal canal via the enlarged neuroforamen (*arrow*).

Intramedullary Tumors

Intramedullary spinal cord tumors constitute only a small fraction of all neoplasms affecting the central nervous system in children, accounting for approximately 6% of cases (34). Their ratio to all the intraspinal tumors is similar to that found in adults, with a value of around 30% (62). However, unlike adults series in which half the patients present with an ependymoma, two thirds of the intramedullary tumors in the pediatric population are astrocytomas (35,62). Indeed, in this age group ependymomas account for only 28.1% of cases; other rare intramedullary tumors include hemangioblastomas, congenital dermoids and epidermoids, as well as non-neoplastic expanding lesions such as syringomyelia and hydromyelia

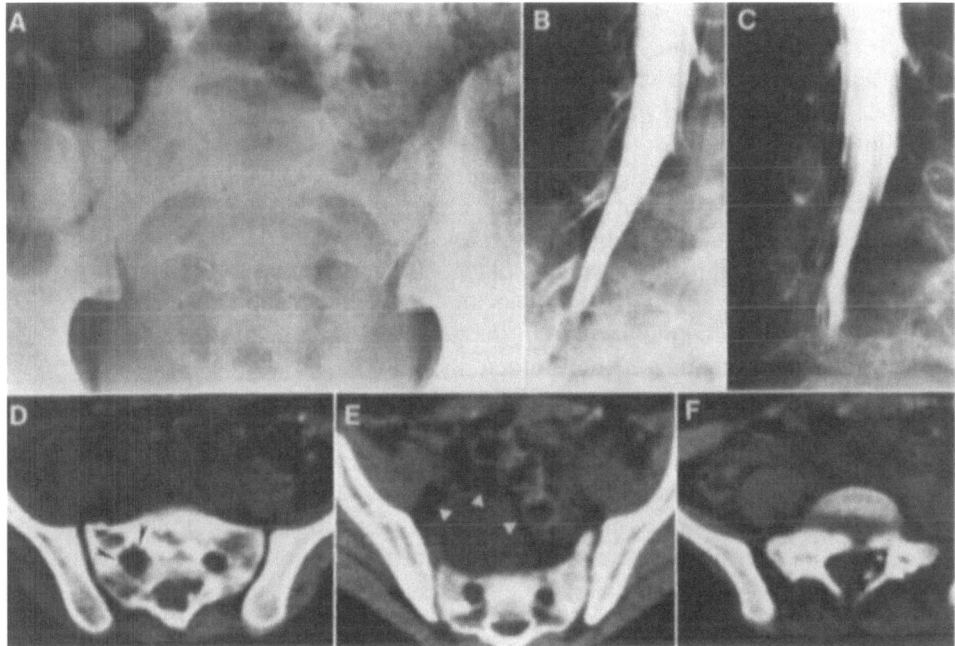

Figure 3.37. Ewing's sarcoma of the sacrum in a 10-year-old boy. **A** Plain film: no obvious bony abnormality of the sacrum. **B,C** Myelogram in oblique (**B**) and sagittal (**C**) projection demonstrates the intraspinal extradural mass from L-5 to S-1. **D,E** Myelo-CT of the sacrum shows the irregular erosion of one left sacral foramen (*black arrowheads* in **D**) and obliteration of the epidural fat within the sacral canal. A round mass bulges in the pelvis from the ventral surface of the left hemisacrum (*white arrowheads* in **E**). **F** Myelo-CT at the L-5 level confirms the intraspinal extradural extension of the tumor: thecal sac is displaced and flattened (*arrowheads*).

(22,35,40,42,49). Intramedullary spinal tumors are equally divided between males and females and show an obvious peak in incidence in children aged from 6 to 15 years.

Two main characteristics distinguish pediatric intramedullary tumors from those in adults: the extension that they can reach before diagnosis, and their prevalence for the rostral segments of the spinal cord (35). In fact, about half of these tumors in children extend over several cord segments, in some cases even involving the entire length of the spinal cord, and two thirds of them are situated in the cervical or cervicothoracic regions. Clinical manifestations of intramedullary tumors do not allow their differential diagnosis with the more common extramedullary tumors; like these, the intramedullary tumors may give symptoms months or even years before their actual discovery. However, exacerbation and remission during the clinical course seem to be particularly common with intramedullary tumors. This phenomenon has been considered related to variations in the peritumoral edema, which are characteristic of this type of neoplasm (3). Similarly, the onset of symptoms, as well as their abrupt worsening after trauma, which is often reported during the course of the disease, has been interpreted as the precipitating effect of an injury to the peritumoral edema (3).

Although pain, which is the frequent presenting symptom of intramedullary tumors, does not provide information that can be utilized for the differential diagnosis of tumors in an extramedullary location, scoliosis as an isolated sign may assume a diagnostic importance. Indeed, in more than half the cases of intramedullary tumors, such an anomaly constitutes the presenting complaint even in the absence of pain. In most children, scoliosis corresponds to the thoracic location of the neoplasm. Head tilt with torticollis and nuchal pain is also relatively common in patients with intramedullary tumors owing to the involvement of the cervical cord segment in more than a third of the cases. In such cases, it is also possible to find the development of an associated hydrocephalus and/or increased intracranial pressure, which are thought to depend on arachnoiditic processes interfering with the normal CSF outflow from the fourth ventricle (3,19).

Neuroradiology of spinal cord intrinsic tumors improved dramatically with the introduction of MRI. Standard X-ray, myelography, intrathecally/ extravenously enhanced CT appear to have little value when compared with MRI.

Conventional evaluation was based on preliminary X-ray films and subsequent myelography and myelo-CT. At conventional radiography one may observe both postural abnormalities (see basic neuroradiology of the spinal mass lesions) and signs of increased "intraspinal pressure." Neither, however, are specific, and, furthermore, the signs of expansile intraspinal lesions are encountered at any level in which there is a spinal cord enlargement (both at the level of the solid tumor and at the levels of the frequently accompanying cysts). Myelography demonstrates directly the extension of the enlarged spinal cord, sometimes with CSF block, but has the same limitations regarding the differential diagnosis of the nodule and of possible associated cysts. Myelo-CT better defines the morphology of the enlarged cord and sometimes allows the late identification of the neoplastic cysts; but this technique requires many repeat serial studies, and demonstration of the cyst is not constant.

Recently one has noted the capability of IVECT in demonstrating abnormal areas of enhancement in intramedullary tumors (63), but the method is extremely uncertain and does not result in a correct definition of the extension of the lesion (which is critical for the surgeon).

Conversely, without any hazards MRI clearly depicts spinal cord expansion, defines the extension and morphology of the tumor, differentiating in most cases cystic from solid components (24,73,80). Generally speaking, when only a cystic expansion is revealed by MRI, the signal intensity of the cyst is the clue to the diagnosis: completely hypodense (like CSF) cysts account for syringo/hydro-myelia, and relatively intense cysts (more intense than CSF in the weighted images) suggest neoplasia (73,95). Currently it is not possible to differentiate between the two most common histotypes of the intramedullary tumor (i.e., astrocytomas and ependymomas). In most cases both tumors exhibit prolonged T1 and T2 values, and one may only assume that an extensive solid tumor is most likely to be an astrocytoma (Fig. 3.38), and a more localized solid unhomogeneous nodule with accompanying upper and lower cysts is more often an ependymoma (Fig. 3.39) (98). The MRI findings may also be influenced by a recent intratumoral hemorrhage, resulting in a shortened T1 and, therefore, high-intensity lesion. Cervical intraspinal extension of a posterior fossa intraaxial tumor is rare, but not exceptional, and MRI is the best-suited method to rule out this feared involvement (Fig. 3.40).

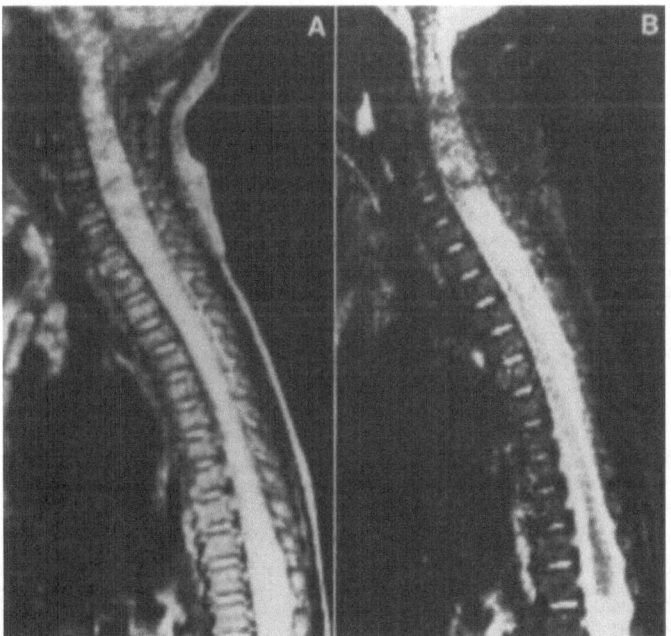

Figure 3.38. Astrocytoma of the cervical cord in a 6-month-old infant. **A** MRI SE; TR-1000, TE-100; **B** MRI SE; TR-1000, TE-200 (heavily T2-weighted). In **A** there is an obvious expansion of the cervical and upper thoracic cord. In **B** the heavily T2-weighted sagittal image discloses a central dishomogeneous nodule (from C-3 to C-6) with high intensity swelling of the cord above and below.

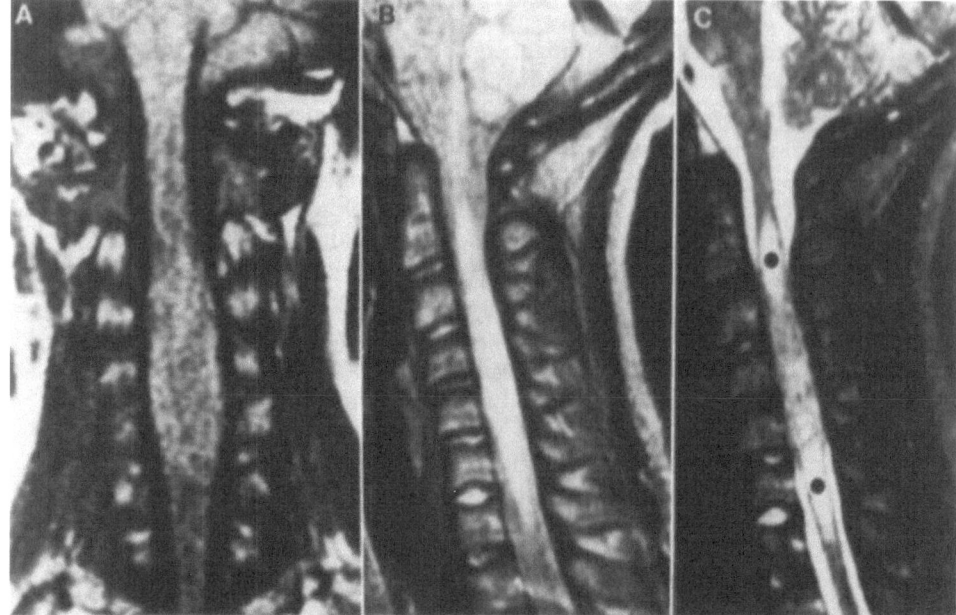

Figure 3.39. Ependymoma of the cervical cord with cyst formation above and below the neoplastic nodule in a 13-year-old girl. **A** MRI, coronal T1-weighted image, demonstrates a mass lesion extending from C-3 to C-6 in the cervical cord with dishomogeneous intensity. At the upper and lower poles of the tumor a relative hypointensity is noted. **B** MRI, sagittal proton density image, optimally depicts the abnormal tissue that exhibits an apparently homogeneous hyperintensity in this sequence. **C** MRI, sagittal heavily T2-weighted image, defines the presence of the solid tumor from C-3 to C-5 with slight hyperintensity. The upper and lower pointed hyperintensities (*black points*) have the same signal of the CSF; this finding suggests cystic dilatation of the central canal. At surgery the accompanying cysts were confirmed, and the tumor was successfully excised.

Astrocytomas

Astrocytomas in pediatric patients are either holocord or focal (34). The "holocord" variety is manifested by an expansion of the entire spinal cord from the medulla or cervicomedullary junction to the conus. It is worth noting that intraspinal astrocytomas rarely go beyond the junction between the spinal cord and brainstem, a characteristic that they share with the corresponding astrocytomas of the cerebellum. Focal astrocytomas are limited expansions of the spinal cord involving several (four to eight) cord segments. The real difference between these two varieties is found in the volume of the associated cystic component, which increases the extension of tumor above and below its solid component along the central spinal canal. The differential diagnosis of cystic astrocytomas ex-

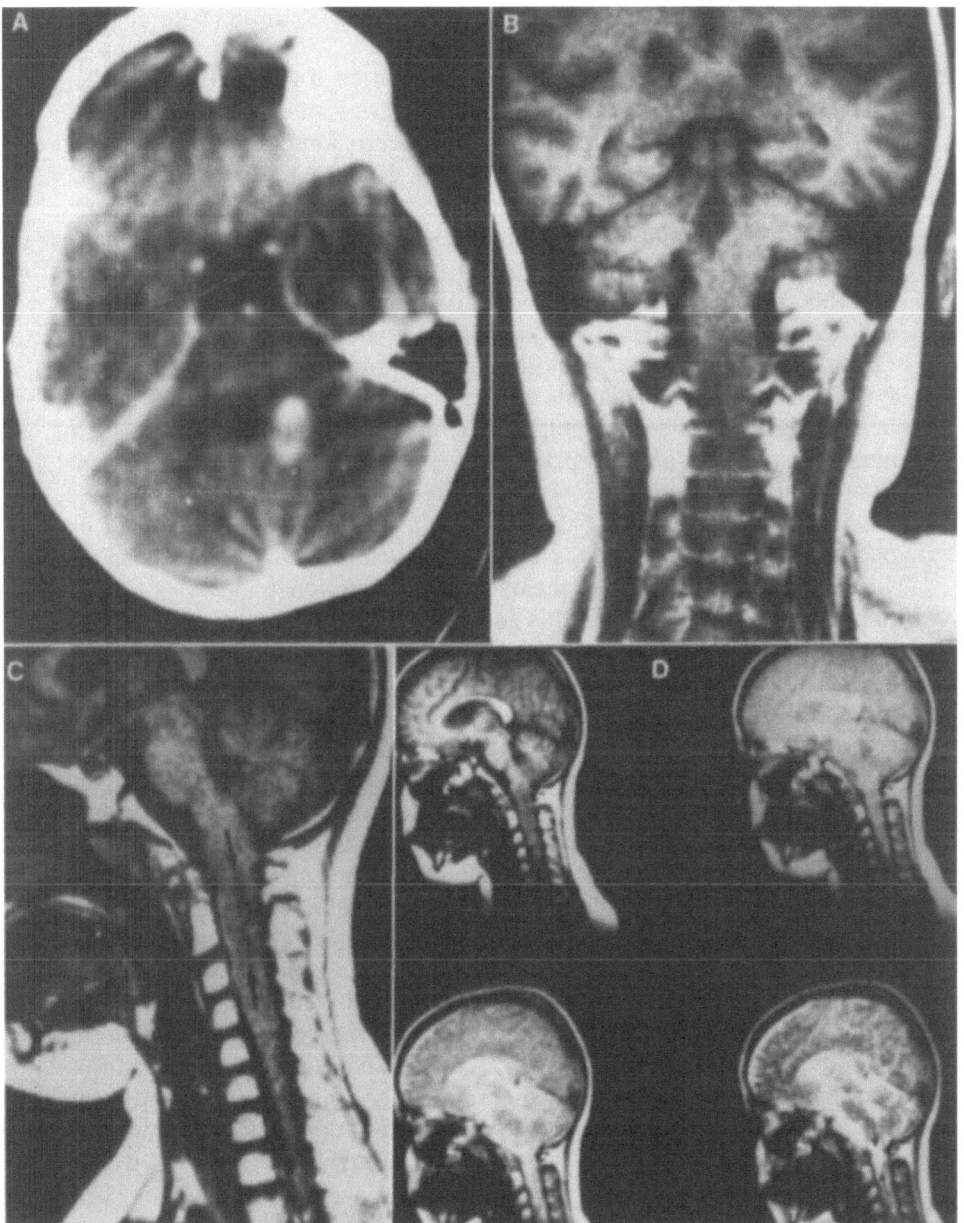

Figure 3.40. Glioma of the hindbrain extending in the cervical cord in a 9-year-old boy. **A** A CT scan shows a small enhancing mass, slightly displacing the fourth ventricle. **B** Coronal T1-weighted image demonstrates the intraxial mass extending through the foramen magnum. **C** Sagittal T1-weighted image depicts the tumor from the fourth ventricle to C-5 with central area of relative hypointensity (*arrows*). **D** Multiecho sagittal SE sequence confirms the extension of the tumor; the central hypointense (*dark)* area becomes hyperintense (*bright*) like CSF in the latest (more T2-weighted) echo suggesting necrosis (*arrows*).

tending for a variable length along the spinal cord with syringomyelia is essentially based on the absence in the latter of an obvious block in the CSF circulation, and on the lack of pedicle erosion due to the expansion of the solid component of the tumor (34). Even in cases of "holocord" astrocytomas, clinical manifestations are directly related to the presence of the solid component, whereas the cystic component remains asymptomatic, at least in the first phases of the disease. It has been hypothesized that this relationship is due to the relatively asymmetrical location of the solid tumoral nodule within the spinal cord, and the paucity of symptoms of the cystic component would be explained by its central location (34). Focal noncystic intramedullary astrocytomas are relatively avascular, grey or pink in color, and distinguishable from the neural tissue; however, in most cases a well-defined plane between the tumor and normal spinal tissue is not apparent, at least on a limited extent of the tumor's surface, where it seems to infiltrate the cord. This area represents the initial implantation of the tumor and is usually characterized by the presence of a vascular pedicle (62). Nevertheless, recent experience indicates that the tumor may be gutted also in this zone, posing an acceptable surgical risk. A posterior midline myelotomy should extend only the length of the actual size of the tumor, and the removal of the lesion should be initiated at its midportion where the astrocytoma usually reaches its maximal volume (97). Also, holocord astrocytomas may be removed with the preservation of the preoperative neurological condition and a relatively long-term cure (35,66,97). The use of intraoperative ultrasonography (90) is particularly helpful in evaluating the extent of the cystic component below and above the solid component. Posterior midline myelotomy should be, in fact, limited to the cord segment above the solid tumoral nodule, its limits being the superior and inferior junctional areas between the cystic and solid components of the astrocytoma. Excision of the solid tumor is initiated at either its caudal or its rostral pole and is facilitated by the lack of adhesion of the anterior surface of the tumor to the cord. In fact, the cyst usually separates the ventral surface of the solid tumor from the normal neural tissue, as the bulk of the tumor usually occupies the posterior two thirds of the spinal cord (97). Holocord astrocytomas should be removed from "inside out" as far as the "glia-tumor interface". This interface is marked by changes in color and consistency, which differentiate if from the adjacent normal neural tissue (97).

Ependymomas

These lesions constitute the second most common intramedullary tumor in children (excluding those at the conus, which are partially intramedullary and partially extramedullary, and those of the filum terminale, which are completely extramedullary). The election site of this tumor, when intramedullary, is the thoracic region. In children, ependymomas grow slowly, sometimes reaching giant proportions before diagnosis. The reason ependymomas may expand for any length of the spinal cord with a relative paucity of signs has been seen in their primarily centred anatomic location in relationship to the central canal. This location would allow the gradual compression of adjacent neural structures, without interfering with the neural functions for a long period of time (97).

Intramedullary ependymomas are frequently associated with cystic or syrinx formations. Encapsulated and relatively avascular ependymomas are usually benign and amenable to surgical resection through a midline incision in the posterior raphe. The presence of a cyst often constitutes a favoring factor by allowing a cleavage plane to be maintained between the tumoral mass and normal neural structures using cottonoid pledgets. The tumor can be shrunk back and drawn away from the cord by coagulating its surface, as well as by necrotizing its core with a bipolar coagulator. The spinal vascular network should be respected, keeping in mind that the perforating branches of the anterior spinal artery usually divide ventrally to the tumor and that the lateral branches supply the spinal cord and the medial branches the tumor (66).

Malignant ependymomas are rare; they are often revealed by their seeding throughout the spinal canal and cranial cavity.

Hemangioblastomas

These neoplasms may occur as isolated lesions or in patients with the von Hippel-Lindau disease (115). Adolescents are preferred (66). Most commonly situated in the cervical or thoracic regions, these tumors are benign, although often highly vascularized. At surgical exploration hemangioblastomas may be seen to reach the external surface of the cord. Usually, these tumors are discrete, extending along only one or two segments of the spinal cord; however, they may be associated with cysts. Surgical excision is favored by moderate vascular hypotension and microsurgical techniques, which allow the progressive "devascularization" of the tumor by progressively coagulating the tumoral blood supply at the interface of the tumor with the surrounding normal neural tissue.

Surgical Considerations

The diagnosis of intraspinal tumors based merely on clinical manifestations is considerably more difficult in children than in adults. Therefore, clinical indications suggestive of this type of lesion should be integrated into the radiographic findings. Plain spine X-ray examination, CT scanning, and MRI make the preoperative localization of the tumor possible in almost all instances, thus allowing surgery to be limited to the minimum required for the complete exposure of the lesion. An early diagnosis is obviously an important favoring factor, as outcomes are generally related to the patient's preoperative status. Before surgery, parents should be informed about the limitations of the surgical procedure and the risk that the operation may actually worsen the clinical condition, as the chronically compressed neural tissue may easily be damaged and the extension of the tumor may be superior to that apparently suggested by the neurological deficits.

The operation is made easier by the use of the operating microscope and modern instrumentation such as the ultrasound surgical aspirator and operating laser. In children the prone position is preferred for almost all lesions. After a midline incision of the skin above the spinous vertebral processes, the spinal exposure should be carried out to encompass fully the extension of the tumor and visualize its rostral and caudal poles. Particular care should be paid in sparing the intervertebral articulations when performing a laminectomy. However, never enough precaution can be taken in children, whose vertebrae are still growing and therefore exposed to the possible development of secondary deformities and instability when undergoing unbalanced mechanical stimulation during physiological maturation. Multiple laminectomies may, in fact, result in the extensive destruction of bone structures and ligaments as well, and the normal laminae and spinous processes are likely to be substituted by scar tissue, onto which the paraspinal muscle masses attach themselves (14). Although in most cases alterations in the statics of the spine resulting from laminectomy cause only moderate disorders in its stability, and these are amenable to orthopedic treatment, in a restricted number of children they may cause neurological functional disasters. Neurological impairment caused directly by the laminectomy mostly occurs in cases of postoperative kyphosis or in patients with scoliosis complicated by relevant deformities occurring in the anteroposterior plane. This type of complication is related to the spinal instability and the age of the patient. The first of these may derive from the tumor itself already in the preoperative phase and from any damage to the intervertebral articulations during operation. Spinal instability is common when the right and left intervertebral articulations have been destroyed at the same level, even when the phenomenon occurs at only one spinal segment (31) (Figs. 3.41, 3.42). The age of the patient is particularly important, as damage to the intervertebral articulations is less frequently followed by kyphosis when the vertebral body is already sufficiently developed in size and mechanical resistance. The development of severe kyphosis is, on the other hand, common in infants under 2 years of age. Furthermore, postoperative spinal alterations tend to worsen with growth, as do all the congenital deformities of the spine. Further intervening factors are the location of the laminectomy (the cervicodorsal and dorsolumbar regions are the most sensitive), the eventually associated radiotherapy (which affects the normal growth of the vertebrae and alone determines characteristic deformities of the vertebral body), and the nature

Figure 3.41. Postlaminectomy deformity with severe increase of the cervical lordosis (same case Fig. 3.20).

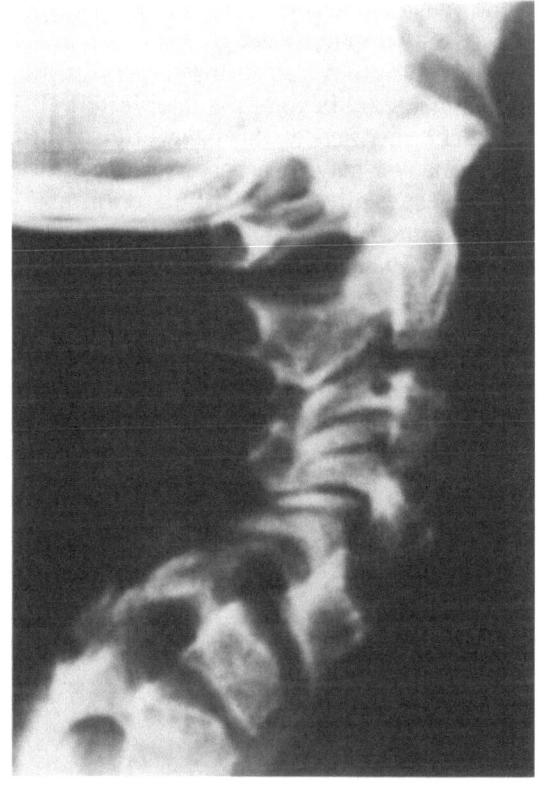

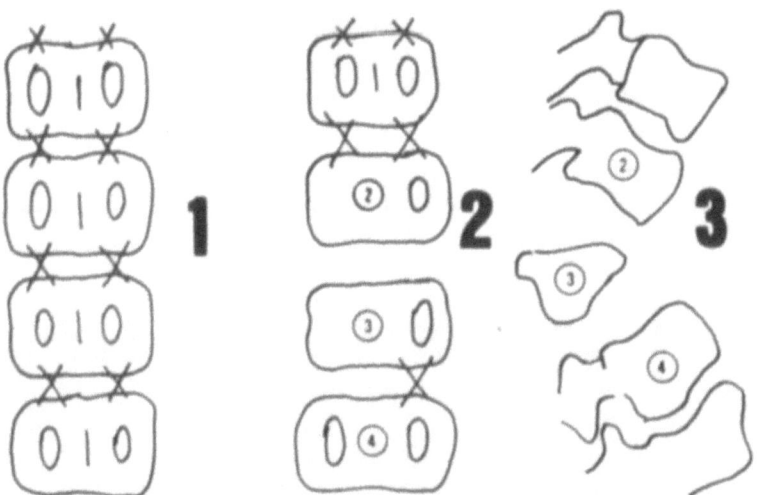

Figure 3.42. Drawing of the postlaminectomy deformity (see text).

of the causative lesion. Conversely, extension of the laminectomy seems to play only a minor role.

Preventive measures during surgery include the avoidance of enlarging the laminectomy beyond the intervertebral articulations and limiting any necessary sacrifice of the intervertebral articulations to only one side. This maneuver may be necessary in cases of intradural but extramedullary tumors, especially dumbbell neurofibromas or meningiomas originating from the anterolateral portions of the dural sac. Postoperative preventive measures consist essentially of orthopedic casts or performing surgical stabilization of the spine.

Laminotomy with anatomical reconstruction of the vertebral arches and reinsertion of interspinous ligaments and paravertebral masses is a valid alternative to laminectomy (91). The technique allows the exposure of any length of the spinal canal without the risk of postoperative spinal deformity or instability. Laminotomy is performed through a laminar osteotomy using a high-speed drill along an imaginary line separating the pedicle from the lamina (Fig. 3.43).

The "laminar" flap, consisting of laminae and intact interspinous and yellow ligaments, is removed in toto, exposing the epidural space to a variable extent. The flap is repositioned and secured with sutures passing through symmetrical drill holes made at either side of the laminotomy incision (Fig. 3.44). Reconstruction is completed by stitching the inter-

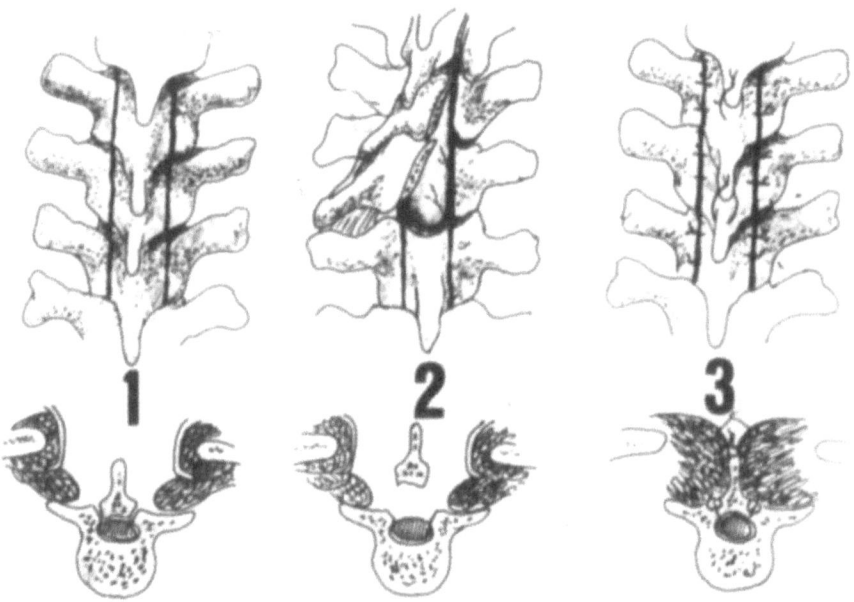

Figure 3.43. Drawing of the laminotomy technique (see text).

Figure 3.44. Radiographic
picture of the postlamino-
tomy state.

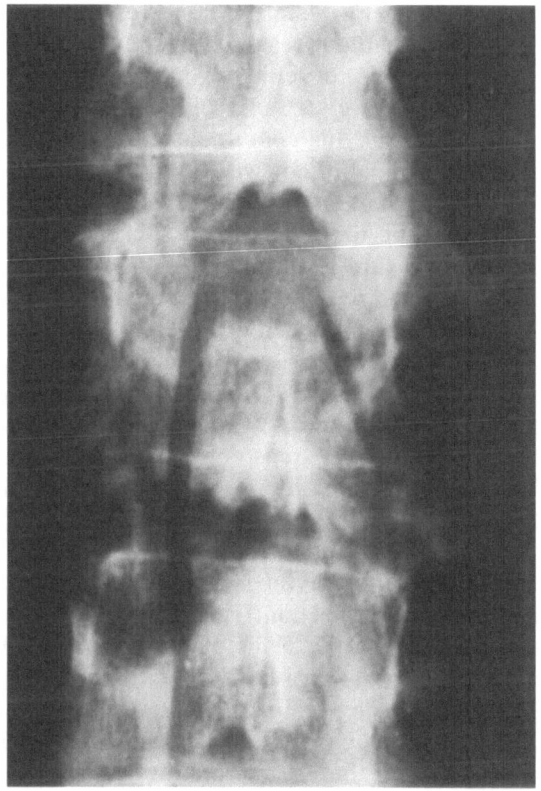

spinous ligaments and paravertebral muscle masses. Appropriate immobilization of the patient with thoracic or lumbosacral casts, or a four-poster
cervical collar according to the spine segment involved, is required after
the operation to ensure postoperative fusion of bone structures.

In removing extramedullary intradural tumors it is necessary to keep
in mind that the spinal cord, although rotatable, turnable, and flexible, is
extremely sensitive to compression, heating, or devascularization (66).
Tension on the cord should be avoided, thus intracapsular decompression
prior to the resection of the tumor should be performed whenever possible.
The maneuver may be facilitated in cases of tumors developing ventrally
or ventrolaterally to the spinal cord, by a transverse cutting of the dura,
and by debulking the tumor out from under the fragile ventral surface of
the cord (106). The vascular supply to the spinal cord should be preserved
in all cases, even when minimal. Ependymomas at the conus medullaris
usually show an exophytic extramedullary component, which should be
removed first. These tumors also develop (intramedullary) within the conus; this portion of the neoplasm should also be removed. The procedure
is often facilitated by a sort of cystic capping, which separates the rostral

end of the tumor from the conus and allows the excision of the tumor from below without resulting in sphincter impairment.

The possibility of removing intramedullary tumors has been known for a long time; however, surgical techniques have improved considerably in the first half of this century. The successful removal of a totally intramedullary spinal tumor was, in fact, first performed by von Eiselberg in 1907 and Elsberg in 1910 (32). Elsberg had inadvertently nicked the cord while opening the dura over a spinal tumor: the accident was followed by the extrusion of the tumoral mass from the cord. The author closed the wound and reexplored the patient one week later, when he discovered that the tumor had been completely extruded from the cord and, consequently, could be easily removed. A second attempt to utilize this two-stage procedure failed (33), but the possibility of the radical removal of intramedullary tumors was subsequently confirmed by other authors (37,84). Significant steps consisted of the introduction of bipolar coagulation and binocular loops (44,45), and, later on, the surgical microscope (92,114).

Intramedullary tumors may be exposed by a midline incision in the posterior raphe after having sealed the crossing vessels with very low-power microbipolar coagulation. The opening of the raphe is then conducted with dissectors along the plane of the perforating vessels. Suction should be adjusted to a minimal level. The tumor is exposed by gently displacing the neural tissue by spreading the tips of the bipolar forceps. The incision in the cord may be kept open by using 7- to 10-monofilament nylon sutures sewn between the pia and the dura. It is worth stressing that careful inspection is necessary before performing the myelotomy, as the cord containing the tumor may be distorted and rotated, and its swelling may have obliterated the posterior median raphe.

The bipolar coagulator is utilized for shrinking the surface of the tumor and coagulating the fine vessels feeding it. Bipolar coagulation is also useful for necrotizing the interior of the tumor, millimeter by millimeter, under saline irrigation (66). A similar maneuver may be carried out using the surgical laser.

The suction-cautery technique can be advantageously substituted by the ultrasonic surgical aspirator, which allows a rapid debulking of the tumoral tissue without transmitting movement to the adjacent neural tissue. Peroperative identification of the solid tumor and its eventual cystic component may be obtained by using ultrasound imaging techniques, generally before opening the dura mater (97).

Finally, sensory-evoked potentials may be monitored throughout the surgical procedure to gather all available information during the operative dissection of the tumor.

Although extensive dissection of the spinal cord may be performed with an acceptable risk, not all the spinal segments offer the same resistance to manipulation. Generally, dissection within the cervical and upper tho-

racic cords, which are largely white matter, is associated with little morbidity, whereas dissections from T-9 to T-12 have the greatest incidence
of postoperative deficits (69). Tumors at the conus usually infiltrate the
gray matter so that the possibility of dissection in this region appears
greatly limited and is invariably followed by sphincter dysfunction.

Among the postoperative complications, wound dehiscence and CSF
fistulas are not rare in children previously subjected to radiotherapy (97).
Of the dural substitutes that can be used in cases of difficult surgical wound
closure, silastic appears to induce minimal reactive fibrosis. Consequently,
the use of silastic has been recommended for cases in which reoperation
is likely (97).

Acknowledgments. The authors are grateful to Professor U. Salvolini,
Chief of the Service of Neuroradiology of the Hospital "Le Torrette" of
Ancona, for having provided some of the figures used in this chapter.

References

1. Andrioli GC, Rigobello L, Iob I, et al.: Multiple meningiomas. Neurochirurgia
   24: 67–69, 1981.
2. Armstrong EA, Harwood-Nash DC, Fitz C, et al.: CT of neuroblastomas
   and ganglioneuromas in children. AJNR 3: 401–406, 1982.
3. Arseni C, Horvath L, Iliescu D: Intraspinal tumours in children. Psychiatr
   Neurol Neurochir 70: 123–133, 1976.
4. Arseni C, Maretsis M: Tumors of the lower spinal cord associated with increased intracranial pressure and papilledema. J Neurosurg 27: 105–110,
   1967.
5. Arthuis M, Turpin JC: Etude clinique des compressions de la moelle et de
   la queue de cheval chez l'enfant, in Rougerie J (ed): Les compressions medullaires non traumatiques de l'enfant. Paris: Masson, 1973, pp 1–20.
6. Aubin ML, Jardin C, Bar D, Vignaud J: CT in 32 cases of intraspinal tumors.
   J Neuroradiol 6: 81–92, 1979.
7. Baleriaux WD, Terwingh G, Jeanmart L: The value of CT in the diagnosis
   of hourglass tumor of the spine. Neuroradiology 14: 31–32, 1972.
8. Banna M, Gryspeerdt GL: Intraspinal tumours in children (excluding dysraphism). Clin Radiol 22: 17–32, 1971.
9. Barnes PD, Lester PD, Yamanashi WS, et al.: Magnetic resonance imaging
   in infants and children with spinal dysraphism. AJNR 7: 468–473, 1986.
10. Batnitzsky S, Keucher TR, Mealey J, et al.: Iatrogenic intraspinal epidermoid
    tumors. JAMA 237: 148–150, 1977.
11. Bradley WG Jr: MRI in the central nervous system: Comparison with
    computed tomography. Magnetic resonance imaging. New York: Raven Press,
    1986, pp 81–122.
12. Brasch RC: MRI for pediatric diagnosis. Magnetic Resonance Annual. New
    York: Raven Press, 1987, pp 179–201.

13. Cairns H, Russell DS: Intracranial and spinal metastases in gliomas of the brain. Brain 54: 377–420, 1931.
14. Cattell HS, Clark GL Jr: Cranial kyphosis and instability following multiple laminectomies in children. J Bone Joint Surg 49A: 713–720, 1967.
15. Chan HSL, Turner-Gomes SO, Chuang SH, et al.: A rare cause of spinal cord compression in childhood from intraspinal mesenchymal chondrosarcoma. Neuroradiology 26: 323–327, 1974.
16. Choremis C, Oeconomos D, Papadatos C, et al.: Intraspinal epidermoid tumors in patients treated for tuberculous meningitis. Lancet 2: 437–439, 1956.
17. Choux M: Lesions kystiques, in Rougerie J (ed): Les compressions medullaires non traumatiques de l'enfant. Paris: Masson, 1973, pp 46–53.
18. Constans JP: Compression extrinsèques malignes, in Rougerie J (ed): Les compressions medullaires non traumatiques de l'enfant. Paris: Masson, 1973, pp 65–76.
19. Coxe WS: Tumors of the spinal canal in children. Am Surg 27: 62–73, 1961.
20. Cramer BC, Jecquier S, O'Gorman AM: Ultrasound of the neonatal craniocervical junction. AJNR 7: 449–457, 1986.
21. Decker R, Gross S: Intraspinal dermoid tumor presenting as chemical meningitis. J Neurosurg 27: 60–62, 1967.
22. De Sousa AL, Kalsbeck JE, Mealey J Jr, et al.: Intraspinal tumors in children: a review of 81 cases. J Neurosurg 51: 437–445, 1979.
23. Deutsch M, Reigel DH: The value of myelography in the management of childhood medulloblastoma. Cancer 45: 2194–2197, 1980.
24. Di Chiro G, Doppman JL, Dwyer AJ, et al.: Tumors and arteriovenous malformations of the spinal cord: assessment using MR. Radiology 156: 689–697, 1985.
25. Di Lorenzo N, Giuffre' R, Fortuna A: Primary spinal neoplasms in childhood: analysis of 1234 published cases (including 56 personal cases) by pathology, sex, age and site. Differences from the situation in adults. Neurochirurgia 25: 153–164, 1982.
26. Di Rocco C, Caldarelli M, Puca A, et al.: Multiple spinal meningiomas in children. Neurochirurgia 27: 25–27, 1984.
27. Djindjian R, Merland JJ: Place de l'embolisation dans le traitement des malformations artério-veneuses medullaires. A propos de 38 cas. Neuroradiology 16: 428–429, 1978.
28. Dorsey J, Tabrisky J: Intraspinal and mediastinal foregut cyst compressing the spinal cord. J Neurosurg 24: 562–567, 1966.
29. Dorwart RH, Masters DL, Watanabe TJ: Tumors, in Newton TH, Potts GD (eds): Modern neuroradiology. San Anselmo: Clavadel Press, 1983, pp 115–147.
30. Dorwart RH, Wara WM, Norman D, et al.: Complete myelographic evaluation of spinal metastases from medulloblastoma. Radiology 1939: 403–408, 1981.
31. Dubousset J, Guillaumat M, Mechin JF: Retentissement rachidien des laminectomies, in Rougerie J (ed): Les compressions medullaires non traumatiques de l'enfant. Paris: Masson, 1973, pp 185–193.
32. Elsberg CA: Diagnosis and treatment of surgical diseases of the spinal cord and its membranes. Philadelphia: WB Saunders Co, 1916, pp 271–281.
33. Elsberg CA: Tumors of the spinal cord. New York: PB Hoeber, 1925, pp 206–239.

34. Epstein F: Spinal cord astrocytomas of childhood. Adv Techn Stand Neurosurg 13: 135–169, 1986.
35. Epstein F, Epstein N: Intramedullary tumors of the spinal cord, in Pediatric neurosurgery. New York: Grune & Stratton, 1982, pp 131–152.
36. Firooznia H, Pinto RS, Lin JL, et al.: Chordoma: radiologic evaluation of 20 cases. AJR 127: 797–805, 1976.
37. Frazier CH: Surgery of the spine and spinal cord. New York: D Appleton, 1918, pp 582–585.
38. Galligioni F: Neuroradiologia. Piccin: Padova, 1980, pp 570–596.
39. Gawehn J, Schroth G, Thron A: The value of paraxial slices in MR imaging of spinal cord disease. Neuroradiology 28: 347–350, 1986.
40. Garrido E, Stein BM: Microsurgical removal of intramedullary spinal cord tumors. Surg Neurol 7: 214–219, 1977.
41. Gibson T, Norris W: Skin fragments removed by injection needles. Lancet 2: 983–985, 1958.
42. Grant FC, Austin GM: The diagnosis, treatment and prognosis of tumors affecting the spinal cord in children. J Neurosurg 13: 535–545, 1956.
43. Graveleau D, De Lopez T, Etienne M, et al.: Tumeurs medullaires du nourisson. Ann Pediatr 41: 439–443, 1965.
44. Greenwood J Jr: Total removal of intramedullary tumors. J Neurosurg 11: 616–621, 1954.
45. Greenwood J Jr: Surgical removal of intramedullary tumors. J Neurosurg 26: 276–282, 1967.
46. Gross RE, Farber S, Martin LW: Neuroblastoma sympateticum. A study and report of 217 cases. Pediatrics 23: 1179–1191, 1959.
47. Grote W, Romer F, Bock WJ, et al.: Langzeitergebnisse in der Behandlung spinaler Tumoren des Kindes- und Jugendalters. Monatsschr Kinderheilkd 123: 112–119, 1975.
48. Guidetti B: Removal of extramedullary benign spinal cord tumors. Adv Techn Stand Neurosurg 1: 173–197, 1974.
49. Haft H, Ransohoff J, Carter S: Spinal cord tumors in children. Pediatrics 23: 1152–1159, 1959.
50. Hahn YS, McLone DG: Pain in children with spinal cord tumors. Childs Brain 11: 36–46, 1984.
51. Hamby WB: Tumour in the spinal canal in childhood. II. Analysis of the literature of a subsequent decade (1933–1942); report of a case of meningitis due to an intramedullary epidermoid communicating with a dermal sinus. J Neuropathol Exp Neurol 3: 397–412, 1944.
52. Harris P: Chronic progressive communicating hydrocephalus due to protein trasudates from brain and spinal tumors. Dev Med Child Neurol 18: 87–94, 1968.
53. Harwood-Nash DC: CT of the pediatric spine: a protocol for the 1980's. Radiol Clin North Am 19: 479–501, 1981.
54. Harwood-Nash DC, Fitz CR: Neuroradiology in infants and children. Saint Louis: CV Mosby Co, 1976, pp 1167–1180.
55. Hendrick EB: Spinal cord tumors in children, in Youmans JR (ed): Neurological surgery. Philadelphia: WB Saunders Co, 1982, pp 3215–3221.
56. Herren P: Papilloma of the choroid plexus. Arch Surg 42: 758–774, 1941.
57. Jequier S, Cramer B, O'Gorman AM: US of the spinal cord in neonates and infants. Ann Radiol 28: 225–231, 1985.

58. Keen C, Coplin A: quoted by Choux: Lesions kystiques, in Rougerie J (ed): Les compressions medullaires non traumatiques de l'enfant. Paris: Masson, 1973, pp 46–53.
59. Kordas M, Paraicz E, Szenasy J: Spinale Tumoren im Säuglings- und Kindesalter. Zentralbl Neurochir 38: 331–338, 1977.
60. Kuchariczyk W, Brandt-Zawadzki M, Sobel D, et al.: Central nervous system tumors in children. Detection by magnetic resonance imaging. Radiology 155: 131–136, 1985.
61. Lachtow RE, L'Hereux PR, Young G, et al.: Neuroblastoma presenting as central nervous system disease. AJNR 3: 623–631, 1982.
62. Laine E, Mansuy L: Tumeurs intra-medullaires, in Rougerie J (ed): Les compressions medullaires non traumatiques de l'enfant. Paris: Masson, 1973, pp 131–152.
63. Lapointe JS, Graeb DA, Nugent RA, et al.: Value of intravenous contrast enhancement in the CT evaluation of intraspinal tumors. AJR 146: 103–107, 1986.
64. Lapras C, Joyeux O, Dechaume JP: Tumeurs des enveloppes, neurinomes et méningiomes, in Rougerie J (ed): Les compressions medullaires non traumatiques de l'enfant. Paris: Masson, 1973, pp 113–130.
65. Lepintre J, Schweisguth D, Labrune M, et al.: Les neuroblastomes en sablier. Etude de vingt-deux cas. Arch Fr Pediatr 26: 829–847, 1969.
66. Malis LI: Intramedullary spinal cord tumors. Clin Neurosurg 25: 512–539, 1978.
67. Manno NJ, Uihlein A, Kernohan J: Intraspinal epidermoids. J Neurosurg 19: 754–756, 1962.
68. Maurice-Williams RS, Lucey JJ: Raised intracranial pressure due to spinal tumors: three rare cases with a probable common mechanism. Br J Surg 62: 92–95, 1975.
69. McArthur R, Fisher R: Aneurysmal bone cyst involving the vertebral column. J Neurosurg 24: 772–776, 1966.
70. McFarland DR, Horwitz H, Saenger EL, et al.: Medulloblastoma: a review of prognosis and survival. Br J Radiol 42: 198–214, 1969.
71. McLaurin RL: Extramedullary spinal tumors, in Pediatric neurosurgery. New York: Grune & Stratton, 1982, pp 541–549.
72. Memon MY, Schneck L: Ventral spinal tumor. The value of CT in its localization. Neurosurgery 8: 108–111, 1981.
73. Modic MT, Mosaryk TJ, Weinstein MA: MRI of the spine, in Magnetic resonance imaging. New York: Raven Press, 1986, pp 55–80.
74. Murad TM, Murthy MSN: Ultrastructure of a chordoma. Cancer 25: 1204–1215, 1970.
75. Naidich TP, McLone DG, Harwood-Nash DC: Spinal dysraphism, in Newton TH, Potts DG (eds): Modern neuroradiology, vol I: CT of the spine and spinal cord. San Anselmo: Clavadel, 1983, pp 299–353.
76. Naidich TP, McLone DG, Shkolnik A, et al.: Sonographic evaluation of the caudal spine and back: Congenital anomalies in children. AJR 142: 1229–1242, 1984.
77. Neil-Dwyer G: Tentorial block of cerebrospinal fluid associated with a lumbar neurofibroma. J Neurosurg 38: 767–770, 1973.
78. Nishio S, Fukui M, Kitamura K, et al.: Intraspinal meningioma in childhood. Childs Brain 8: 382–389, 1981.

79. Nittner K: Raumbeengende Prozesse im Spinalkanal, in Olivecrona H, Tonnis W, Krinkel W (eds): Handbuch der Neurochirurgie, vol 2. New York: Springer-Verlag, 1972, pp 1–606.
80. Norman D: The spine, in Brant-Zawadzki M, Norman D (eds): Magnetic resonance of the central nervous system. New York: Raven Press, 1987, pp 289–328.
81. Occhipinti E, Mastrostefano R, Pompili A, et al.: Spinal chordomas in infancy: report of a case and analysis of the literature. Childs Brain 8: 198–206, 1981.
82. Oi S, Raimondi AJ: Hydrocephalus associated with intraspinal neoplasms in childhood. Am J Dis Child 135: 1122–1124, 1981.
83. Pena CE, Horvat BL, Fisher ER: The ultrastructure of chordoma. Am J Clin Pathol 53: 544–551, 1970.
84. Poppen JL: An Atlas of Neurosurgical Techniques. Philadelphia: WB Saunders Co, 1960, p 424.
85. Porras CL: Meningioma in the forame magnum in a boy aged 8 years. J Neurosurg 20: 167–168, 1963.
86. Portela LA: Sonography of the normal and abnormal intact lumbar spinal canal. AJNR 5: 791–795, 1984.
87. Post MJD, Quencer MR, Green BA, et al.: Intramedullary spinal cord metastases, mainly of non neurogenic origin. AJNR 8: 339–346, 1987.
88. Quencer RM, Montalvo BM: Normal intraoperative spinal sonography. AJR 143: 1301–1306, 1984.
89. Quencer RM, Montalvo BM, Naidich TP, et al.: Intraoperative sonography in spinal dysraphism and syringomyelia. AJNR 8: 329–338, 1987.
90. Raghavendra BN, Epstein FJ, McCleary L: Intrameduallary spinal cord tumors in children: localization by intraoperative sonography. AJNR 5: 395–397, 1984.
91. Raimondi AJ, Gutierrez FA, Di Rocco C: Laminotomy and total reconstruction of the posterior spinal arch for spinal canal surgery in childhood, J Neurosurg 45: 555–560, 1976.
92. Rand RW: Microneurosurgery. St. Louis: CV Mosby Co, 1969, pp 210–214.
93. Rand RW, Rand CW: Intraspinal Tumors of Childhood. Springfield: Charles C Thomas Publisher, 1960.
94. Richè MC, Melki JP, Merland JJ: Embolization of spinal cord vascular malformations via the anterior spinal artery. AJNR 4: 378–381, 1983.
95. Rubin JM, Aisen AM, Di Pietro MA: Ambiguities in MR imaging of tumoral cysts in the spinal cord. J Comput Assist Tomogr 10: 395–398, 1986.
96. Schiffer J, Mundel G, Lahat E, et al.: Multiple meningiomas in separate neuroaxial compartments in a child. Childs Brain 6: 287–288, 1980.
97. Schijman E, Zuccaro G, Monges JA: Spinal tumors and hydrocephalus. Childs Brain 8: 401–405, 1981.
98. Scotti G, Scialfa G, Colombo N, et al.: Magnetic resonance diagnosis of intramedullary tumors. Neuroradiology 29: 130–135, 1987.
99. Scotti G, Scialfa G, Landoni L: MR imaging of intradural extramedullary tumors of the cervical spine. J Comput Assist Tomogr 9: 1037–1041, 1985.
100. Shapiro R: Myelography. Year Book Publishers, ed 3. 1973, pp 143–198.
101. Shaywitz B: Epidermoid spinal cord tumors and previous lumbar punctures. J Pediatr 80: 638–640, 1972.
102. Siegel MJ, Jamroz GA, Glazer HS, et al.: MR imaging of intraspinal extension of neuroblastoma. J Comput Assist Tomogr 10: 593–595, 1986.

103. Simpson D: The recurrence of intracranial meningiomas after surgical treatment. J Neurol Neurosurg Psychiatry 20: 22–39, 1957.
104. Smoker WRK, Biller J, Moore SA, et al.: Intradural spinal teratoma: Case report and review of the literature. AJNR 7: 905–910, 1986.
105. Stanley P, Senac MO Jr, Segall HD: Intraspinal seeding from intracranial tumors in children. AJR 144: 157–161, 1985.
106. Stein B: Spinal intradural tumors, in Wilkins RH, Rengachary SS (eds): Neurosurgery. New York: McGraw-Hill Book Co, 1985, pp 1048–1061.
107. Stern WE: Localization and diagnosis of spinal cord tumors. Clin Neurosurg 25: 480–494, 1978.
108. Suit HD, Goiten M, Munzenrider J, et al.: Definitive radiation therapy for chordoma and chondrosarcoma of the base of skull and cervical spine. J Neurosurg 56: 377–385, 1982.
109. Svien JH, Gates EM, Kernohan JW: Spinal subarachnoid implantation associated with ependymoma. Arch Neurol Psychiatry 62: 847–856, 1949.
110. Svien JH, Mabon RF, Kernohan JW, et al.: Ependymoma of the brain: pathological aspects. Neurology (NY) 3: 1–15, 1953.
111. Van Gilder JG, Schwartz HG: Growth of dermoids from skin implants to nervous system and surrounding spaces of newborn rat. J Neurosurg 26: 14–20, 1967.
112. Vittini F: Kystes épidermoides et dermoides, les tératomes kystiques, in Rougerie J (ed): Les compressions medullaires non traumatiques de l'enfant. Paris: Masson, 1973, pp 40–46.
113. Wilhyde D, Jane J, Mullan S: Spinal epidural leukemia. Am J Med 34: 281–287, 1963.
114. Yasargil G: Microsurgery applied to neurosurgery. Stuttgart: Thieme-Verlag, 1969, pp 175–177.
115. Yasargil MG, Antic J, Laciga R, et al.: The microsurgical removal of intramedullary spinal hemangioblastomas: report of twelve cases and a review of the literature. Surg Neurol 6: 141–148, 1976.

CHAPTER 4

Nonoperative Treatment of Tumors of the Spinal Cord in Children

Samuel Neff and R. Michael Scott

Introduction

It is generally agreed that primary therapy for spinal cord tumors should consist of complete surgical excision. In most cases modern operative neurosurgical techniques can achieve this. In cases where surgical excision is incomplete, where the tumor is inherently diffuse, or in recurrent disease, nonoperative therapy must be employed.

General Concepts

Radiation therapy, chemotherapy, and immunotherapy have all shown in vitro activity against central nervous system (CNS) tumors. Clinically, radiotherapy and chemotherapy of spinal cord tumors have been studied sporadically. Because of the relative rarity of these tumors in the pediatric age group, many principles of therapy must be extrapolated from experience with brain tumors of similar histology in adults.

Radiation Therapy

Conventional radiation therapy for spinal cord tumors consists of high-energy photons in the form of x-rays or gamma rays (102). The biological effects of photon irradiation have been comprehensively reviewed (44) and, in particular, the long-term effects on the CNS have been studied (1,22,64,74,94,100,110).

High-energy radiation in the form of particle beams holds certain theoretical advantages over conventional techniques (12,13,37,46,90,103); the application of these methods to spinal cord tumors is the subject of current investigations (90,98).

Radiation therapy for the pediatric spinal cord is limited by direct myelotoxicity and radiation-induced vasculopathy (100,110). As with radiation therapy to the brain, direct toxicity to neurons and glia is determined by total dose and fractionation schedule (1). Additional factors unique to spinal cord are length and section irradiated, with some evidence from studies in adults suggesting that different segments have differing tolerances (1,58,78). The clinical significance of secondary toxicity due to vasculopathy is not clear. Research is hampered by a paucity of autopsy series, the impracticality of tissue biopsy, the added myelotoxic effects of chemotherapy and recurrent tumor (56), and the variable interval between radiation and pathologic examination (18,35). In general, dosage and fractionation schedules to achieve a maximum therapeutic ratio have been derived by extrapolation from experience with brain irradiation, except in common tumors such as medulloblastoma.

Long-term follow-up of children treated with neuraxis radiation has shown growth arrest at the epiphyseal plates (51). This was originally interpreted as a direct effect of radiation to the immature vertebral column (22,74,82). Recently, it has been shown that this represents the effect of a reduction in growth hormone secretion secondary to whole-brain (therefore anterior pituitary) radiation (2,20,94,107). A correlation exists between age at time of treatment and ultimate height loss, with younger children having more severe effects (95). Treatment with growth hormone is effective and not associated with increased tumor growth or relapse (17). Radiation-induced tumors have not been associated with dose levels employed in the treatment of pediatric spinal cord tumors (44,51), but a recent report suggests that if follow-up times are sufficiently long a small number will be seen (72).

Chemotherapy

Chemotherapy is assuming increasing importance in the treatment of pediatric spinal cord tumors. In addition to standard protocols for metastatic tumors, trials have been reported for intrinsic CNS neoplasms. These are discussed under individual tumors below. The toxicity of intrathecal chemotherapy has not been extensively studied except in conjunction with radiation therapy, where combination of both modalities may permit lower doses (62,71).

The biochemistry of chemotherapy for spinal cord tumors is entirely analogous to that described for CNS tumors in general. Intra-arterial chemotherapy is not currently used in treating spinal cord tumors because of the complex vascular anatomy of the spinal cord. Phase I trails must await clear demonstration of efficacy in more accessible CNS tumors.

Immunotherapy

Immunotherapy holds great promise as an adjuvant therapy for CNS tumors. At present there have been no reports of its use in tumors of the pediatric spine.

Primary Spinal Cord Tumors

Astrocytoma

In the pediatric population astrocytomas constitute 55% to 60% of intra-medullary spinal cord tumors (26,32). In addition, intracranial astrocytomas may disseminate to the leptomeninges (16). Prolonged survival has been seen after complete resection, after incomplete resection, and after biopsy without radiotherapy (23).

In cases where gross total excision of low-grade spinal cord astrocytomas was performed, adjunctive radiotherapy was administered routinely, selectively (54), or not at all (26,27) with both prolonged survival and rapid recurrence seen in all three groups. This variability has led to a search for predictors of outcome. Histology correlates with overall survival but not clearly with radiosensitivity.

The long-term results of microsurgical excision of low-grade spinal cord astrocytomas are not known. Radiotherapy should therefore be limited to incompletely excised or recurrent, unresectable lesions. The radiated port should include all involved segments of the cord as determined by modern diagnostic testing [computed tomography (CT) myelograms, intraoperative ultrasonography, or nuclear magnetic resonance (NMR) tomography]. No controlled trials of radiation therapy have been reported for spinal cord astrocytomas. Recommended maximum dosage in adults is 4,000 rad with a 10% reduction for the thoracic region (57). Radiation myelopathy has been reported in children receiving as little as 3,000 rad ' to the spinal cord (100). As a result, radiation dosage in children is generally held below this level.

High-grade astrocytomas of the spinal cord constitute a significant fraction of astrocytomas in the pediatric age group (25,66). These tumors are locally aggressive despite local radiotherapy, but have shown no tendency to metastasize to distant regions (55). Therapy thus consists of biopsy and radiation to cord tolerance at the involved segments. Available clinical data show a survival advantage with conventional whole-neuraxis radiotherapy. The use of chemotherapy must be considered experimental (60,61).

Oligodendroglioma

Oligodendroglioma is a rare tumor of the pediatric spinal cord, constituting less than 1% of reported cases (19,23). No information is available on the long-term prognosis or effects of various treatment modalities. Radiation therapy should be reserved for incompletely resected lesions.

Meningioma

These tumors constitute less than 4% of spinal cord tumors in children (23). Therapy consists of surgical excision. There is no demonstated role for radiation therapy.

Medulloblastoma

Treatment of primary medulloblastoma with craniospinal axis radiation therapy and chemotherapy as outlined in modern protocols, may or may not include maintenance chemotherapy (6,11,53,68,83,104).

Recurrent medulloblastoma involves the spinal cord in 12% of all cases (40,77). Standard treatment is chemotherapy; radiation therapy is given if sufficiently localized disease is found (7,20,84). Since unsuccessfully treated recurrence results in death from systemic metastatic disease (69), some degree of myelotoxicity may be tolerated. The toxicities of chemotherapeutic agents are at least additive to that of radiotherapy (18).

Several protocols for recurrent medulloblastoma have been reported. In one report (63), 36 cases of recurrent medulloblastoma were treated with aggressive chemotherapeutic regimens including ara-C (cytosine arabinoside), methotrexate and thio-TEPA administered by direct subarachnoid injection; CCNU (lomustine) procarbazine, vincristine, and dianhydrogalactitol systemically. Some patients received radiation therapy with misonidazole sensitization. This series was conducted while chemotherapeutic regimens were evolving, so patients received a variable combination of treatments. A more recent study (29) reported experience with 143 consecutive cases of medulloblastoma. The addition of chemotherapy did not result in a significant increase in survival over surgery and radiation alone. No firm conclusions about the effectiveness of chemotherapy can be drawn from the data. Controlled clinical trials are underway using more advanced protocols (10).

Ependymoma

Primary ependymomas constitute 25% to 30% of spinal cord tumors in the pediatric age group (23,24). In addition, a small fraction of patients with ependymoma presenting above the foramen magnum will go on to develop clinical spinal metastases (65); an incidence of 30% was seen in one autopsy series (101).

Postoperative radiation therapy for ependymoma has not been studied in a prospective randomized fashion, although ependymomas are radiosensitive (96). Retrospective studies have varied, some treating all cases with craniospinal axis irradiation (65), with other authors recommending treatment for selected cases (96).

A consensus exists that long-term results are dependent on the location and grade of tumor, with the character of adjuvant therapy, if any, assuming secondary importance. With documented spinal metastasis, 3,000 to 4,000 rad to the entire spinal axis is recommended, with a reduction for children less than 3 years old (88,89).

The myxopapillary ependymomas of the filum terminale constitute up to 50% (14) of spinal ependymomas. Radiation with a total dose of 4,500 to 5,000 rad in 180 to 200-rad fractions has been recommended (14,33); however, long-term survival, despite late recurrence, has been reported with subtotal resection and lower doses (93) or without radiation (111). Nevertheless, in the absence of controlled studies, it is reasonable to administer radiation unless microscopic complete excision is achieved (97). Intracranial metastasis has been reported in adults only (21).

Treatment results with metastatic ependymoma are uniformly poor (106). Chemotherapy for ependymoma has been reported (106), but must be considered experimental.

Chordoma

Chordomas constitute 0.7% of all CNS tumors (76). They are locally aggressive and have metastatic potential. Only 13 cases of spinal (vertebral) chordomas have been reported in the pediatric age group (76,86,99). In the ten patients whose therapy was stated, six received surgery only; one received radiotherapy only; two received surgery and radiotherapy; and one received surgery, radiotherapy, and chemotherapy. The three long-term (greater than 1 year) survivors are two patients disease free at 4 and 15 years after treatment with surgery only, and one patient with persistent disease at 4 years after treatment with radiotherapy only. Similar long-term palliation is achieved in adult chordoma cases (50,91). No conclusions about the effectiveness of nonoperative therapy can be made. Complete surgical removal constitutes the only proven curative therapy.

Primary CNS Lymphoma

This lymphoma involving the spinal cord constituted less than 3% of pediatric spinal cord tumors in one series (23) and accounted for none in 80 cases of another series (45). Treatment consists of radiation (43) or radiation and intrathecal chemotherapy (64). Spinal cord dosage is 3,500 rad with a 1,000-rad boost to areas of bulky disease (49,59). Chemotherapeutic agents administered include high-dose methotrexate and intrathecal methotrexate with or without alternating ara-C, cyclophosphamide, vincristine, and prednisone. There is insufficient evidence to recommend a particular protocol, and patients should be entered in a controlled trial if possible.

Ganglioglioma

There are four reported cases of spinal gangliogliomas in children (3,34,48). All patients are alive at 4 months to 14 years after diagnosis without evidence of recurrence. Because of the benign nature of this neoplasm, radiotherapy and chemotherapy are not recommended.

Epithelial Cysts

Epidermoid and dermoid tumors constituted 10% of pediatric spinal cord tumors in two series (23,38). These tumors present as expanding mass lesions because of the secretory and desquamation products of the tumor epithelium. With modern surgical techniques, complete resection is the rule. With incomplete resection, regrowth is often extremely slow and adjuvant therapy is not recommended.

Sacrococcygeal Teratoma

Sacrococcygeal teratoma occurs at a rate of 1 in 40,000 births, with an 80% female predominance (30). Primary treatment consists of surgical excision. The role of adjuvant radiation and chemotherapy in incompletely excised tumors is unclear (85), although improved survival was seen in one uncontrolled trial (4).

Metastasis from Systemic Neoplasms

Neuroblastoma

Neuroblastoma constitutes 5% to 20% of pediatric intraspinal tumors overall (23,39), and an even greater fraction in infants (5). Approximately 20% of neuroblastomas involve the vertebral column (105). Central nervous system involvement occurs almost exclusively by direct invasion (112).

Surgery alone has not been proved effective for primary treatment of advanced-stage neuroblastoma (28,80). Spinal cord compression can be relieved by surgical decompression or radiotherapy (23,79). Treatment with aggressive chemotherapeutic regimens and radiation has improved survival in children less than 1 year old, with less effect on survival in older age groups (28,31,36,42,75,79,92).

Neuroblastoma is radiosensitive, and palliation or local control can be achieved with external beam therapy. Doses ranging from 2,500 to 2,750 rad are employed for microsopic disease; for gross residual tumor doses are increased to 2,750 to 3,250 rad. Recently, low-dose therapy ranging from 900 to 1,500 rad has been shown to be effective (47).

Various protocols have employed whole-body radiotherapy in conjuction with chemotherapy, although one study demonstrated no effect (36).

Experimental protocols, including high-dose radiation and chemotherapy with autologous bone marrow rescue, are currently in progress. The limiting toxicity of these regimens is often bone marrow suppression, and autologous bone marrow rescue would be employed except that more than half of spinal neuroblastoma involves the bone marrow at presentation. Current research is directed toward eliminating neuroblastoma from the autologous bone marrow in vitro using monoclonal antibodies (81).

Wilm's Tumor

Wilm's tumor is the second most common non-CNS solid tumor in children. Overall, Wilm's tumor involves the spine or spinal cord in 1% of reported cases (9). Before initial surgery, chemotherapy may be administered to reduce tumor bulk (79,108). Postoperative radiation therapy is administered if vertebral spread is not resected completely or in the presence of hematogenous metastases, although the optimal dosage has not been determined (79). In two reported cases of spinal cord involvement, treatment consisted of standard chemotherapeutic protocols and local radiation therapy to cord tolerance (9). The results obtained with adjuvant chemotherapy and radiation therapy in the National Wilm's Tumor Study showed no benefit in achieving gross total excision at the expense of vital organ function. The neurosurgeon confronted with spinal cord compression should thus perform an adequate surgical decompression and not attempt removal of all microscopic tumor.

Malignant Tumors of Bone

Osteogenic Sarcoma

Osteogenic sarcoma constitues 3.1% of pediatric solid tumors. In one series metastatic disease involved the spinal cord by epidural compression in seven of 16 cases (87). Treatment consisted of irradiation and chemotherapy with methotrexate/folinic acid, doxorubicin, and cyclophosphamide. All patients had relief of pain, and objective radiologic response was documented in six of seven patients with bone lesions.

Ewing's Sarcoma

The second most common bone tumor in childhood is Ewing's sarcoma, accounting for 2% of all malignancies in children (79). The fraction (8%) involving the vertebral column constitutes approximately 10% of spinal cord sarcomas in children. Intradural metastasis has been reported (109), but is much less common than extradural disease (70).

The tumor is responsive to radiation alone, as well as to cyclophosphamide, doxorubicin, vincristine, BCNU (carmustine), and other single agents (79). Phase I trials of single-agent chemotherapy showed frequent relapse; therefore, a cooperative trial of combination chemotherapy and radiation was begun (73). Radiation consisted of 4,500 to 5,500 rad in 200-rad fractions with a 100-rad boost to bulky tumor with soft-tissue extension; all patients received vincristine, actinomycin, and cyclophosphamide. Patients who received the above with the addition of doxorubicin had a 2-year survival of 72%. Further improvement in survival has been demonstrated using cyclophosphamide, doxorubicin, vincristine, actinomycin

D, and BCNU in a study where some patients received no radiation (41). In contrast, total-body irradiation has been associated with excellent outcome in some reports (52). High-dose total-body irradiation with autologous bone marrow rescue, systemic chemotherapy, and local radiation resulted in induction of remission in 90% of cases in one series (79). Selective irradiation of either the upper- or lower-halfbody followed at 5 weeks by irradiation of the other half has been associated with improved long-term survival (8).

Sarcomas of Soft-Tissue Origin

Rhabdomyosarcoma

Paraspinal rhabdomyosarcoma constitutes 5% to 7% of all rhabdomyosarcomas, which, in turn, make up 3.7% of pediatric neoplasms (79). In the First Intergroup Rhabdomyosarcoma Study, improved survival was associated with gross total surgical removal and nonalveolar histology. When total removal is achieved with negative resection margins, local radiation therapy is not indicated. When examination of resection margins demonstates microscopic residual disease, conventional radiation therapy of 5,000 rad has been recommended. Bulky residual disease should be aggressively treated with interstitial brachytherapy or electron beam. All patients with rhabdomyosarcoma should receive adjuvant chemotherapy appropriate for the stage disease. These are set forth in the report of the Second Intergroup Rhabdomyosarcoma Study (67).

Chondrosarcoma

Overall, chondrosarcoma is a rare tumor, and only 3.8% of cases occur in the pediatric population (15). Treatment consists of surgical excision. Radiation therapy probably retards the progress of the tumor; nevertheless, most treatment failures are local recurrences. Therapy for residual or unresectable tumor should consist of the highest radiation dose tolerated by the spinal cord. Chemotherapy has not been reported to be effective.

Conclusion

In studies performed to date, diagnosis of spinal cord tumors has relied primarily on clinical evaluation and invasive diagnostic tests, particularly myelography. New diagnostic tests, particularly NMR and CT, have revolutionized the diagnosis and management of spinal cord tumors. By permitting noninvasive imaging of the cord and surrounding structures, these techniques have made it possible to monitor the extent of residual disease and screen for recurrence on a routine basis. When these imaging techniques become more widely available, precise determination of the efficacy of radiation and chemotherapy in these tumors will be possible.

Immunotherapy, radiation sensitizers, and hyperthermia are currently being explored for use in CNS neoplasms. The application of these techniques to spinal cord tumors awaits further research.

References

1. Abbatucci JS, Delozier T, Quint R, et al.: Radiation myelopathy of the cervical spinal cord: Time, dose, and volume factors. Int J Radiat Oncol Biol Phys 4:239–248, 1978.
2. Albertsson-Wikland K, Lannering B, Marky I, et al.: A longitudinal study on growth and spontaneous growth hormone (GH) secretion in children with irradiated brain tumors. Acta Paediatr Scand 76:966–973, 1987.
3. Albright L, Byrd RP: Ganglioglioma of the entire spinal cord. Childs Brain 6:274–280, 1980.
4. Applebaum H, Exelby PR, Wollner N: Malignant presacral teratoma in children. J Pediatr Surg 14:352–355, 1979.
5. Balakrishnan V Rice MS Simpson DA: Spinal neuroblastomas. J Neurosurg 40:631–638, 1974.
6. Bellani FF, Gasparini M, Lombardi F, et al.: Medulloblastoma: Results of a sequential combined treatment. Cancer 54:1956–1961, 1984.
7. Berry MP, Jenkin RD, Keen CW, et al: Radiation treatment for medulloblastoma: A 21-year review. J Neurosurg 55:43–51, 1981.
8. Berry MP, Jenkin RDT, Harwood AR, et al.: Ewing's sarcoma: A trial of adjuvant chemotherapy and sequential half-body irradiation. Int J Radiat Oncol Biol Phys 12:19–24, 1986.
9. Bever CT Jr, Koenigsberger MR, Antunes JL, et al.: Epidural metastasis by Wilm's tumor. Am J Dis Child. 135:644–646, 1981.
10. Bloom HJG: Medulloblastoma in children: increasing survival rates and further prospects. Int J Radiat Oncol Biol Phys 8:2023–2027, 1982.
11. Brown RC, Gunderson L, Plenk HP: Medulloblastoma. A review of the LDS hospital experience. Cancer 40:56–60, 1977.
12. Castro JR, Quivey JM, Lyman JT, et al.: Current status of clinical particle radiotherapy at Lawrence Berkeley Laboratory, Cancer 46:633–641, 1980.
13. Castro JR, Saunder WM, Tobias CA, et al.: Treatment of cancer with heavy charged particles. Int J Radiat Oncol Biol Phys 8:2191–2198, 1982.
14. Chan HS, Becker LE, Hoffman HJ, et al.: Mxyopapillary ependymoma of the filum terminale and cauda equina in childhood: report of seven cases and review of the literature. Neurosurgery 14:204–210, 1984.
15. Chan HS, Turner Gomes SO, Chuang SH, et al.: A rare cause of spinal cord compression in childhood from intraspinal mesenchymal chondrosarcoma. A report of two cases and review of the literature. Neuroradiology 26:323–327, 1984.
16. Civitello LA, Packer RJ, Rorke LB, et al.: Leptomeningeal dissemination of low-grade gliomas in childhood. Neurology 38:562–566, 1988.
17. Clayton PE, Shalet SM, Gattamaneni HR, Price DA: Does growth hormone cause relapse of brain tumours? Lancet 1 (8535):711–713, 1987.

18. Cohen ME, Duffner PK, Terplan KL: Myelopathy with severe structural derangement associated with combined modality therapy. Cancer 52:1590–1596, 1983.

19. Coxe WS: Tumors of the spinal canal in children. Am Surg 27:62–73, 1961.

20. Cumberlin RL, Luk KH, Wara WM, et al.: Medulloblastoma: treatment results and effect on normal tissues. Cancer 43:1014–1020, 1979.

21. Davis C, Barnard RO: Malignant behavior of myxopapillary ependymoma. J Neurosurg 62:925–929, 1985.

22. Dawson WB: Growth impairment following radiotherapy in childhood. Clin Radiol 19:241–256, 1968.

23. DeSousa AL, Kalsbeck JE, Mealey J Jr et al.: Intraspinal tumors in children: a review of 81 cases. J Neurosurg 51:437–445, 1979.

24. Dohrmann GJ, Farwell JR, Flannery JT: Ependymomas and ependymoblastomas in children. J Neurosurg 45:273–283, 1976.

25. Epstein F: Spinal cord astrocytomas in children. Adv Tech Stand Neurosurg 13:136–169, 1986.

26. Epstein F, Epstein N: Surgical management of holocord intramedullary spinal cord astrocytomas in children: Report of three cases. J Neurosurg 54:829–832, 1981.

27. Epstein F, Epstein N: Surgical treatment of spinal cord astrocytomas of childhood. J Neurosurg 57:685–689, 1982.

28. Evans AE, D'Angio GJ, Koop CE: The role of multimodal therapy in patients with local and regional neuroblastoma. J Pediatr Surg 19:77–80, 1984.

29. Farwell JR, Dohrmann GJ, Flannery JT: Medulloblastoma in childhood: an epidemiological study. J Neurosurg 61:657–664, 1984.

30. Filston HC: Sacrococcygeal teratomas, in Wilkins RH, Rengachary SS (eds): Neurosurgery. New York: McGraw-Hill Co, 1985.

31. Finkelstein JZ, Klemperer MF, Evans A, et al.: Multiagent chemotherapy for children with metastatic neuroblastoma: A report from CCSG. Med Pediatr Oncol 6:179–188, 1979.

32. Garcia DM: Primary spinal cord tumors treated with surgery and postoperative irradiation. Int J Radiat Oncol Biol Phys 11:1933–1939, 1985.

33. Garrett PG, Simpson WJ: Ependymomas: results of radiation treatment. Int J Radiat Oncol Biol Phys 9:1121–1124, 1983.

34. Garrido E, Becker LE, Hoffman HJ, et al.: Gangliogliomas in children. Childs Brain 4:339–346, 1978.

35. Godwin-Austen RB, Howell DA, Worthington B: Observations on radiation myelopathy. Brain 98:557–568, 1975.

36. Green MA, Hustu HO, Palmer R, et al.: Total body sequential segmented irradiation and combination chemotherapy for children with disseminated neuroblastoma. Cancer 38:2250–2257, 1976.

37. Griffin TW, Laramore GE, Hussey DH, et al.: Fast neutron beam radiation therapy in the United States. Int J Radiat Oncol Biol Phys 8:2165–2168, 1982.

38. Guttierez FA, Sizuo O, McLone D: Concepts in pediatric neurosurgery, vol 4. Basel: Karger, 1983, pp 291–305.

39. Haft H, Ransohoff J, Carter S: Spinal cord tumors in children. Pediatrics 23:1152–1159, 1959.

40. Harisiadis L, Chang CH: Medulloblastoma in children: a correlation between

staging and results of treatment. Int J Radiat Oncol Biol Phys 2:833–841, 1977.

41. Hayes FA, Thompson EI, Hustu HO, et al.: The response of Ewing's sarcoma to sequential cyclophosphamide and Adriamycin induction therapy. J Clin Oncol 1:45–51, 1983.

42. Hayes FA, Green AA, Casper J, et al.: Clinical evaluation of sequentially scheduled cis-platinum and VP-26 in neuroblastoma: Response and toxicity. Cancer 48:1715–1718, 1981.

43. Helle TL, Britt RH, Colby TV: Primary lymphoma of the central nervous system. Clinicopathological study of experience at Stanford. J Neurosurg 60:94–103, 1984.

44. Hellman S: Principles of radiation therapy, in DeVita VT, Hellman S, Rosenberg SA (eds): Cancer, 2 ed. Philadelphia: JB Lippincott Co, 1985.

45. Hendrick EB: Spinal cord tumors in children, in Youmans JR (ed): Neurological surgery, 2 ed. Philadelphia: W B Saunders Co, 1982.

46. Hornsey S, Morris CC, Myers R, et al.: Relative biological effectiveness for damage to the central nervous system by neutrons. Int J Radiat Oncol Biol Phys 7:185–189, 1981.

47. Jocobson HM, Marcus RB, Thar TL, et al.: Pediatric neuroblastoma: postoperative radiation therapy using less than 2000 rad. Int J Radiat Oncol Biol Phys 9:501–505, 1983.

48. Johannsson JH, Rekate HL, Roessman U: Gangliogliomas: pathological and clinical correlation. J Neurosurg 54:58–63, 1981.

49. Jones GR, Mason WH, Fishman LS, et al.: Primary central nervous system lymphoma without intracranial mass in a child. Cancer 56:2804–2808, 1985.

50. Karakousis CP, Park JJ, Fleminger R, et al.: Chordomas: Diagnosis and management. Am Surg 47:497–501, 1981.

51. Katzman H, Waugh T, Berdon W: Skeletal changes following irradiation of childhood tumors. J Bone Joint Surg [Am] 51A:825–842, 1969.

52. Kinsella TJ, Glaubiger D, Diesseroth A, et al.: Intensive combined modality therapy including low dose TBI in high risk Ewing's sarcoma patients. Int J Radiat Oncol Biol Phys 9:1955–1960, 1983.

53. Kopelson G, linggood RM, Kleinman GM: Medulloblastoma. The identification of prognostic subgroups and implication for multimodality management. Cancer 51:312–319, 1983.

54. Kopelson G, Linggood RM, Kleinman GM, et al.: Management of intramedullary spinal cord tumors. Radiology 135:473–479, 1980.

55. Kopelson G, Linggood R: Infratentorial glioblastoma: the role of neuraxis irradiation. Int J Radiat Oncol Biol Phys 8:999–1003, 1982.

56. Kopelson G: Radiation tolerance of the spinal cord previously damaged by tumor and operation: long term improvement and time-dose-volume relationships after irradiation of intraspinal gliomas. Int J Radiat Oncol Biol Phys 8:925–929, 1982.

57. Kramer S: Complications of radiation therapy - the central nervous system. Semin Roentgenol 9:75–83, 1974.

58. Lambert PM: Radiation myelopathy of the thoracic spinal cord in long term survivors treated with radical radiotherapy using conventional fractionation. Cancer 41:1751–1760, 1978.

59. Leavens ME, Manning JT, Wallace S, et al.: Primary lymphoma of the central

nervous system, in Wilkins RH, Rengachary SS (eds): Neurosurgery. New York: McGraw-Hill Co, 1985.

60. Lefkowitz IB, Packer RJ, Sutton LN, et al.: Results of the treatment of children with recurrent gliomas with lomustine and vincristine. Cancer 61:896–902, 1988.

61. Levin VA, Chamberlain MC, Prados MD, et al.: Phase I-II study of eflornithine and mitoguazone combined in the treatment of recurrent primary brain tumors. Cancer Treat Rep 71:459–464, 1987.

62. Levin VA, Rodriguez LA, Edwards MS, et al.: Treatment of medulloblastoma with procarbazine, hydroxyurea, and reduced radiation doses to whole brain and spine. J Neurosurg 68:383–387, 1988.

63. Levin VA, Vestnys PS, Edwards MS, et al.: Improvement in survival produced by sequential therapies in the treatment of recurrent medulloblastoma. Cancer 51:1364–1370, 1983.

64. Loeffler JS, Ervin TJ, Mauch P, et al.: Primary lymphomas of the central nervous system: patterns of failure and factors that influence survival. J Clin Oncol 3:490–494, 1985.

65. Marks JE, Adler SJ: A comparative study of ependymomas by site of origin. Int J Radiat Oncol Biol Phys 8:37–43, 1982.

66. Marsa GW, Goffinet DR, Rubinstein LJ, et al.: Megavoltage irradiation in the treatment of gliomas of the brain and spinal cord. Cancer 36:1681–1689, 1975.

67. Maurer HM, Moon TE, Donaldson M, et al.: The Intergroup Rhabdomyosarcoma study. Cancer 40:2015–2026, 1977.

68. McIntosh S, Chen M, Sartain PA, et al.: Adjuvant chemotherapy for medulloblastoma. Cancer 56:1316–1319, 1985.

69. Mealey J Jr, Hall PV: Medulloblastoma in children. Survival and treatment. J Neurosurg 46:56–64, 1977.

70. Mehta Y, Hendrickson FR: CNS involvement in Ewing's sarcoma. Cancer 33:859–862, 1974.

71. Moss HA, Nannis ED, Poplack DG: The effects of prophyllactic treatment of the central nervous system on the intellectual functioning of children with acute lymphocytic leukemia. Am J Med 71:47–52, 1981.

72. Moss SD, Rockswold GL, Chou SN, et al.: Radiation-induced meningiomas in pediatric patients. Neurosurgery 22:758–761, 1988.

73. Nesbit ME, Perez CA, Tefft M, et al.: Multimodal therapy for the management of primary nonmetastatic Ewing's sarcoma of bone: An intergroup study. Natl Cancer Inst Monogr 56:255–262, 1981.

74. Neuhauser EBD, Wittenborg MH, Berman CZ, et al.: Irradiation effects of roentgen therapy on the growing spine. Radiology 59:637–650, 1952.

75. Nitschke R, Starling K, Lui VKS, et al.: Doxorubicin and cisplatin therapy in children with neuroblastoma resistant to conventional therapy: A Southwest Oncology Group Study. Cancer Treat Rep 65:1105–1108, 1981.

76. Occhipinti E, Mastrostefano R, Pompili A, et al.: Spinal chordomas in infancy: Report of a case and analysis of the literature. Childs Brain 8:198–206, 1981.

77. Park TS, Hoffman HJ, Hendrick EB, et al.: Medulloblastoma: clinical presentation and management. Experience at the Hospital for Sick Children, Toronto, 1950–1980. J Neurosurg 58:543–552, 1983.

78. Phillips TL, Sheline GE, Boldey E: Therapeutic considerations in tumors affecting the central nervous system: Ependymomas. Radiology 83:98–105, 1964.
79. Pizzo PA, Cassady JR, Miser JS, et al.: Solid tumors of childhood, in DeVita VT, Hellman S, Rosenberg SA (eds): Cancer, 2 ed. Philadelphia: J B Lippincott Co, 1985.
80. Priebe C, Clatworthy H: Neuroblastoma, evaluation of the treatment of 90 children. Arch Surg 95:538–545, 1967.
81. Pritchard J, McElwain TJ, Graham-Pole J: High dose melphalan with autologous marrow for treatment of advanced neuroblastoma. Br J Cancer 45:86–94, 1982.
82. Probert JC, Parker BR, Kaplan HS: Growth retardation in children after megavoltage irradiation of the spine. Cancer 32:634–639, 1973.
83. Quest DO, Brisman R, Antunes JL, et al: Period of risk for recurrence in medulloblastoma. J Neurosurg 48:159–163, 1978.
84. Raimondi AJ, Tomita T: Medulloblastoma in childhood: comparative results of partial and total resection. Childs Brain 5:310–328, 1979.
85. Raney RB, Chatten J, Littman P, et al.: Treatment strategies for infants with malignant sacrococcygeal teratoma. J Pediatr Surg 16:573–577, 1981.
86. Reddy EK, Mansfield CM, Hartman GV: Chordoma. Int J Radiat Oncol Biol Phys 7:1709–1711, 1981.
87. Rosen G, Tefft M, Martinez A, et al.: Combination chemotherapy and radiation therapy in the treatment of metastatic osteogenic sarcoma. Cancer 35:622–630, 1975.
88. Salazar OM, Castro Vita H, VanHoutte P, et al.: Improved survival in cases of intracranial ependymoma after radiation therapy. Late report and recommendations. J Neurosurg 59:652–659, 1983.
89. Salazar OM: A better understanding of CNS seeding and a brighter outlook for postoperatively irradiated patients with ependymomas, Int J Radiat Oncol Biol Phys 9:1231–1234, 1983.
90. Saunders WM, Castro JR, Chen GTY, et al.: Early results of ion beam radiation therapy for sacral chordoma. J Neurosurg 64:243–247, 1986.
91. Saxton JP: Chordoma. Int J Radiat Oncol Biol Phys 7:913–915, 1981.
92. Schuster JJ, Land VJ, Nitschke R, et al.: Phase II study of four-drug chemotherapy for metastatic neuroblastoma: A Pediatric Oncology Group Study. Cancer Treat Rep 67:187–188, 1983.
93. Scott M: Infiltrating ependymomas of the cauda equina: Treatment by conservative surgery plus radiotherapy. J Neurosurg 41:446–448, 1974.
94. Shalet SM, Beardwell CG, Pearson D, et al.: The effects of varying doses of cerebral irradiation on growth hormone production in childhood. Clin Endocrinol 5:287–290, 1976.
95. Shalet SM, Gibson B, Swindell R, et al.: Effect of spinal irradiation on growth. Arch Dis Child 62:461–464, 1987.
96. Shuman R, Alvord E, Leech R: The biology of childhood ependymomas. Arch Neurol 32:731–739, 1975.
97. Sonneland PR, Scheithauer BW, Onofrio BM: Myxopapillary ependymoma. A clinicopathologic and immunocytochemical study of 77 cases. Cancer 56:883–893, 1985.
98. Suit HD, Goitein M, Munzenrider J, et al.: Definitive radiation therapy for

chordoma and chondrosarcoma of base of skull and cervical spine. J Neurosurg 56:377–385, 1982.

99. Sundaresan N, Galicich JH, Chu FC, et al.: Spinal chordomas. J Neurosurg 50:312–319, 1979.

100. Sundaresan N, Gutierrez FA, Larsen MB: Radiation myelopathy in children. Ann Neurol 4:47–50, 1978.

101. Svien H, Gates E: Spinal subarachnoid implanation associated with ependymoma. Arch Neurol Psychiatr 62:847–856, 1949.

102. Tefft M, Mitus A, Schulz MD: Initial high dose irradiation for metastases causing spinal cord compression in children. Am J Roentgenol Radium Ther Nucl Med 106:385–393, 1969.

103. Tobias CA, Blakely EA, Alpen EL, et al.: Molecular and cellular radiobiology of heavy ions. Int J Radiat Oncol Biol Phys 8:2109–2120, 1982.

104. Tomita T, McLone DG: Medulloblastoma in childhood: results of radical resection and low-dose neuraxis radiation therapy. J Neurosurg 64:238–242, 1986.

105. Traggis DG, Filler RM, Druckman H, et al.: Prognosis for children with neuroblastoma presenting with paralysis. J Pediatr Surg 12:419–425, 1977.

106. Van Eys J, Chen T, Moore T, et al.: Adjuvant chemotherapy for medulloblastoma and ependymoma using IV vincristine, intrathecal methotrexate, and intrathecal hydrocortisone: A Southwest Oncology Group Study. Cancer Treat Rep 65:681–684, 1981.

107. Venes JL: Concepts in pediatric neurosurgery, vol 2. Basel: Karger, 1982, pp 1–13.

108. Wagner CW, Parrish RA: Use of preoperative chemotherapy and radiation therapy in patients with Wilms' tumors. Ann Surg 47:190–194, 1981.

109. Wald SL, Roland TA: Intradural spinal metastasis in Ewing's sarcoma: case report and review of the literature. Neurosurgery 15:873–877, 1984.

110. Wara, WM, Phillips TL, Sheline GE, et al.: Radiation tolerance of the spinal cord. Cancer 35:1558–1562, 1975.

111. Wight DGD, Holley KJ, Finbow JAH: Metastasizing ependymoma of the cauda equina. J Clin Pathol 26:929–935, 1973.

112. de la Monte SM, Moore GW, Hutchins GM: Nonrandom distribution of metastases in neuroblastic tumors. Cancer 52:915–925, 1983.

CHAPTER 5

Surgical Considerations for Access to the Spinal Canal

Anthony J. Raimondi

It is not possible to state realistically what the single most important aspect of an operative procedure is (diagnosis, anatomic localization, blood control, exposure, body position). However, it is possible to state that if the surgeon positions the child's body properly, taking into consideration the location of the lesion and the planned skin incision, he will, throughout the operation, be oriented anatomically and always have the lesion at the center of his operative field.

Positioning for pediatric neurosurgery varies considerably with the age of the child (newborn, infant, toddler, juvenile); number of surgeons (one surgeon alone, surgeon and assistant, etc.); location of the anesthesiologist and amount of monitoring equipment; and target area.

Within limits, none of these considerations applies to neurosurgical operative procedures on adolescents or adults, since the patient is uniform in size, and there are no anatomical considerations, such as presence of ossification centers, that assume primary importance. Therefore, this chapter presents to the reader general and specific considerations concerning age, individual body positions, and relative position of the surgeon vis-à-vis the patient (1).

Considerations on Positioning of the Operating Miscroscope, Laser, MEP, and Echo for Intraoperative Use

The positioning of the operating microscope for intraoperative use is variable, ranging from those neurosurgeons who always position the microscope in the same place in the operating room and then accommodate themselves and position the child around the microscope base and arms, to those who use highly mobile floor- or ceiling-mounted microscopes that may be adapted, albeit with considerable effort, to the child throughout the operative procedure. Valid points may be made for either. The author prefers the latter, since it provides greater range of motion and superior utilization of the instrument. Different anatomical locations of surgical lesions in childhood demand a versatile, highly mobile operating micro-scope.

The operating table and chair should be so designed as to complement one another, allowing the surgeon to adjust automatically the position of either vis-à-vis the other, irrespective of the position of the child. Although the best designed surgeon's chair may provide a greater degree of comfort and a lesser degree of fatigability, the closer the chair position approxi-mates normal sitting posture, the longer the surgeon will be able to operate without tiring. When it is necessary to extend the chair from the phys-iological sitting posture into one that more closely resembles a high stool with arm rests, fatigue occurs more quickly. The ceiling-mounted micro-scope may be easily and quickly adjusted so as to permit one to operate on a patient in either the horizontal or the sitting position, without en-cumbering the floor space or readjusting the positions of the anesthe-siologist, neurophysiologist, and the nurses.

Both laser and echo units are large, floor-mounted, awkward, and dif-ficult to manipulate. However, the benefits that each provides the surgeon are well worth the encumbrance, fatigue, and effort. Each operating room and each procedure are so very different from one another that it is mean-ingless to attempt to provide detailed guidelines for the use of these in-struments. Very likely, advances in technology will considerably simplify the laser, echo, and multivariant-evoked potential (MEP) recordings, al-lowing the former to be used with ease through the operating microscope and resulting in the development of a much smaller "head" for effective use of the latter. They are all very expensive, delicate, highly technical instruments that necessitate training in their use. The MEP requires an experienced neurophysiologist.

Regardless of the kind of laser used (e.g., carbon dioxide, argon, neo-dymium YAG, etc.), the beam may be delivered to the target area by using either a hand-held device or by mounting a micromanipulator to the operating microscope.

Intraoperative MEPs provide supportive data concerning functional in-tegrity of the visual somatosensory or auditory and brain stem conductive pathways.

Laminotomy

The prone position is ideal for cervical, thoracic, and lumbar laminotomies:

a) Cervical laminotomy: Maximum exposure of the cervical spine and spinal cord is obtained by positioning the child prone in identically the same manner as for inferior cerebellar triangle exposure through suboc-cipital craniotomy. This brings the inion into a position that does not ob-struct the surgeon's line of vision to the atlas, permits him entry into the posterior foass if needed, and gives him a very complete and direct view of the entire cervical cord.

b) Thoracic laminotomy: For upper thoracic laminotomies it is best to place the head in a neutral position, distracting it only slightly, but not turning it to either side, depending exclusively on the preference of the surgeon and anesthesiologist. Turning of the head to one side or the other with child prone rotates the cervical vertebrae on one another, so that one may encounter rotation of C-7 on T-1. This is the reason for distracting the head and keeping it in a neutral position for upper thoracic laminotomy.

c) Lumbar laminotomy: This requires the simplest positioning of any neurosurgical procedure. The head may be turned to either side and the child (children of all ages) need only be placed prone with rolls and pillows beneath the shoulders, and beneath the shoulders and iliac crests in toddlers, juveniles, and adolescents.

Multiple-level laminectomies are an acceptable surgical approach to spinal cord lesions in adults but not in young children. In most adult patients the procedure is not followed by instability of the spine. In children, however, multiple-level laminectomies cause kyphosis, scoliosis, anterior subluxation, and instability of the cervical, thoracic, or lumbar spines. Physiological anatomy resulting from laminectomy and laminotomy are discussed later under those headings, respectively.

The *draping* is simple and paramedian, exposing the sagittal plane and 2 cm laterally on either side.

The *skin incision* is midline, extending the full length of the planned laminotomy plus 4 cm cephalad and 4 cm caudad. If one is operating or a neuroma that extends into both the spinal canal and the retropleural or retroperitoneal spaces, a "hockey-stick" incision is ideal. Its short limb is placed over the spinous processes, the long limb extended, with a curvilinear arch, over the rib cage or abdominal wall.

Several structures provide for the stability of the spinal column: intervertebral joints, laminae, ligamentum flavae, spinous processes, inter-spinous and supraspinous ligaments, and paraspinal muscles. In the adult, stability depends mostly on the intervertebral joints, and the role of the other structures is relatively less important. The vertebrae of the child are developing structures for which balanced mechanical stimulations are necessary to ensure normal growth. Spinal deformity and/or instability result from conditions in which bone and ligamentous deficiencies or neuromuscular imbalances occur. Such conditions may be caused by multiple laminectomies that destroy growing bony structures (laminae and spinous processes), separate interlaminar and interspinous ligaments from adjoining vertebral arches, and *substitute scar tissue for insertion of paraspinal muscle masses onto the laminae and spinous processes.*

After the skin incision has been made and clips applied to the subcutaneous connective tissue, the thin paraspinous muscles are cut from their insertion along the midline of the vertebral arch and then stripped free.

Muscle and ligamentous attachments are separated from the spinal arches, leaving the periosteum and interspinous ligaments intact. The dissection is carried laterally to just beyond the articular facets, with care being taken not to open into the joint or strip the capsular ligaments.

The closure is facilitated if one leaves a ruffle of muscle and ligament on the spinal apophyses. In newborn and infants, there is no, or very little, spinous process, and the laminae are both narrow and thin. The paraspinous muscle masses are minuscule. Hence, one should use a small periosteal elevator to separate the paravertebral muscles from the vertebral arches, which are immediately encountered on making the incision.

For the closure, the paraspinous muscles are allowed to fall into place by removing the self-retaining retractor. Then, the muscles are sewed down to the interspinous ligaments of the anchored laminar flap as well as to those above and below the laminotomy. This reapproximates the paraspinous muscles, interspinous ligaments, spinous processes, and laminae, restoring anatomical continuity between them. This reapproximation is probably responsible for avoiding the postoperative scoliosis so commonly observed in children with laminectomy for spinal cord surgery, since it assures uniform muscular pull on the spinal column after healing has been completed. Postoperative scoliosis is uncommon following laminotomy. The skin over the spinal column is closed with mattress sutures.

Laminectomy is a destructive procedure that is indicated when there are intraspinal metastases compressing the cord or cauda equina. When the intraspinal pathology is traumatic, benign neoplastic, or congenital malformation (eg, diastematomyelia, diplomyelia, dermoid sinus tract), laminectomy may further weaken the spinal column. Decompressive laminectomy for the drainage of epidural tuberculous abscess makes subsequent fusion—the treatment of choice—difficult for impossible. Whenever a limited or extensive laminectomy (two or more levels) is performed on a child, kyphosis and scoliosis may develop and become difficult clinical problems, necessitating spinal fusion. Kyphosis, anterior subluxation, and instability of the spine are postoperative complications of multiple-level laminectomies in children. The surgical procedure of multiple-level laminotomies is the preferable alternative.

Scoliosis and kyphosis following multiple-level laminectomies in children were described in 1965 by Tachdjian and Matson (2) and then confirmed in 1967 by Cattell and Clark (3). In 1955 Bette and Englehardt (4), were the first to point out that anterior intervertebral body subluxation and kyphosis occurred following laminectomy. Since these changes have not been observed in adults, one must conclude that there is a fundamental anatomical and physioanatomical difference between the fully developed and completely grown vertebral spine and the developing, nonossifed spine of younger children (infants, toddlers, juveniles). In addition, one must take into consideration the complete development of the paraspinal muscle masses in the adult, and the underdeveloped and nonfunctional erector spinae masses in the infant.

In their 1967 paper, Cattell and Clark noted that Tachdjian and Matson failed to comment on whether their 24 patients with cervical cord lesions developed cervical column instability, whereas they elaborated on the onset of scoliosis and kyphosis at the thoracic and lumbar levels following multiple laminectomies in 115 children. This concerned Cattell and Clark, who were particularly interested in the fact that the cervical spine, the most mobile segment of the vertebral column, was especially subject to the destabilizing effects of laminectomy. They demostrated that skeletal, ligamentous neuromuscular, and progressive bony growth (with ossification of the centra) were all, to a greater or lesser degree, responsible for vertebral column deformity following laminectomy. One of the most important points that these authors make is that the vertebrae in children are dynamic, growing and ossifying, structures which, most important of all, offer purchase to developing muscle masses. They concluded that abnormal growth patterns and greater elasticity of musculoligamentous structures in children are responsible for the rapid and severe deformities of the vertebral column, especially the cervical column, which result following laminectomy.

Following the work of Raimondi et al. (5), which concluded that deformities (kyphosis, scoliosis, accentuated lordosis) of the vertebral column in childhood result from laminectomy and which recommended that laminotomy be substituted for laminectomy, Yasuoka et al (6) reported that "postlaminectomy spinal deformity can develop in children without irradiation or facet injury." Yasuoka et al. concluded that deformity results from a wedging transformation of the cartilaginous component of the vertebral bodies and that increased viscoelasticity of children's musculoligamentous structures is a significant contributory factor. Their attention was directed primarily to the treatment of postlaminectomy deformities of the vertebral column in childhood, not to abandoning the laminectomy and adapting laminotomy as the procedure of choice for access to the spinal canal in childhood.

On this subject an important contribution to the literature was made by Barbera et al. (7) who reported on their study of the "laminectomy membrane," previously described by La Rocca and Macnab (8). Specifically, the laminectomy membrane was found to be pathogenetic in producing or reproducing signs and symptoms of spinal cord compression following a laminectomy procedure. The laminectomy membrane is nothing more than scar tissue. Barbera et al. recommended using either an acrylic plastic or kiel bone graft over the dura mater to prevent "expansion of the scar tissue inside the spinal canal and adhesions between the dura and the cicatricial overlying muscles." They concluded that this type of solid material, or tissue, is necessary to prevent the formation of the "laminectomy membrane."

Laminotomy, consequently, (a) restores bony protection to the spinal cord, (b) prevents or significantly diminishes postoperative spinal column deformity (kyphosis, accentuated lordosis, scoliosis), and (c) eliminates the formation of a laminectomy membrane.

Criteria for performing a laminotomy include the extent of the surgical procedure, the age of the patient, and the nature of the lesion. In children under 1 year of age one should perform a laminotomy even if only one level is to be exposed; in children between 1 and 15 years old, for two or more levels; and in patients older than 15 years when three or more levels are to be exposed. Independent of the patient's age or of the extent of the intraspinal lesion, laminotomy should be performed in all patients with trauma, syringomyelia, hydromyelia, or tuberculosis. No attempt should be made to perform laminotomy in children with extensive epidural metastases.

Several structures provide for the stability of the spinal column: intervertebral joints, laminae, ligamentum flavum, spinous processes, interspinous and supraspinous ligaments, and paraspinal muscles. In the adult, stability depends mostly on the intervertebral joints, and the role of the other structures of the posterior arch is relatively less important. The vertebrae of the child are developing structures for which balanced mechanical stimulations are necessary to ensure normal growth. Spinal deformity and/ or instability result from conditions in which bone, ligamentous deficiencies, or neuromuscular imbalance, occur. Such a condition results from multiple laminectomies, which destroy growing bony structures (laminae and spinous processes), separate interlaminar and interspinous ligaments from adjoining vertebral arches, and substitute scar tissue for insertion of paraspinal muscle masses onto the laminae and spinous processes.

The reflection of a free laminar flap (9, 10) over the intraspinal pathology allows as complete access to the spinal canal as the most extensive laminectomy, since the lateral border of the laminotomy is at the medial surface of the pedicle. Multiple-level laminotomy flaps provide access to the entire spinal canal (C-1 through T-3, T-5 through L-3, L-2 through L-5), thereby allowing surgical removal of the most extensive lesions without weakening permantly the vertebral column or destroying the growth center in the posterior portion of the spinal arch.

The removal of multiple laminae in a single laminar flap is a tedious procedure, and requires considerably more time than a laminectomy. It is not a more dangerous procedure than laminectomy, since magnification and high-speed drills permit one to separate the laminae and yellow ligaments with precision.

Performance of a laminotomy instead of a laminectomy permits complete reconstruction of the posterior arch of the spinal canal and *significantly diminishes* the complication of postlaminectomy scoliosis. It provides for complete anatomical reconstruction of the dura, the posterior arch of the spinal canal, and the muscular-bone relationships between the erector spinae muscles on one hand and the spinous processes and interspinous ligaments on the other.

Procedure

After the midline skin incision has been made and extended the desired length, the skin is reflected laterally. The dissection is then carried along the midline using the electrocautery knife (never the laser in young children). Care must be taken to remain within the ligamentous, structures between one spinous process and another until coming upon the tips of the spinous processes.

The exposure should extend from one full vertebra above through one full vertebra below the planned extent of the laminotomy. Thus, if a laminar flap is to be reflected from C-3 through T-4, one should expose the laminae from C-2 through T-5. Muscle and ligamentous attachments are separated from the vertebral arches, leaving the periosteum and interspinous ligaments intact. The dissection is carried laterally to just beyond the articular facets, with care being taken not to open into the joint or to strip the capsular ligaments. The closure is facilitated if one leaves a ruffle of muscle and ligament on the spinous apophyses.

The younger the child, the smaller the spinous processes and the thinner the laminae. Similarly, the younger the child the thinner the erector spinae muscle mass. In fact, in the newborn and infant the spinous processes are almost nonexistent so that the laminae form a rather "domelike" structure. In muscle and bone development the infant is intermediate, between the newborn and the toddler. Since the relative sizes of the laminae and yellow ligaments are eequal, there is no shingling effect of the superior laminae overlapping the inferior laminae. This shingling occurs at approximately 6 to 10 years of age, when the muscle masses begin to develop. Once the spinous processes and laminae have been cleaned of adherent muscle and fascia, one may proceed to perform the laminotomy.

The laser is currently being used more and more in neurological surgery, and since it is ideal for dissecting erector spinae muscles from the spinous processes and laminae in the adult, it deserves comment at this time. *Its use in spinal cord injury and in children with spinal cord tumors is to be recommended when the child is over 10 years of age, but to be avoided completely when the child is under 5 years of age.* The exception is dissection of paraspinous muscles in children with spina bifida aperta upon whom a kyphectomy is being performed. Its use in the 5 to 10 year old is to be decided upon only after computed tomography (CT) scans and x-ray studies of the spinal column reveal that the spinous processes are completely formed and that the laminae are thick and overlap one another. This care must be taken since the laser beam may penetrate the yellow ligaments and dura as the surgeon is dissecting the muscles from the laminae, with the resultant risk of damaging spinal nerves or the spinal cord. Since the newborn and infant have yellow ligaments that are almost as wide as the laminae, one readily understands the risk. In the older child thick, overlapping laminae completely protect the dura and the cord.

The respective inferior and superior yellow ligaments are then incised from medial to lateral, bilaterally, prior to proceeding with the laminar osteotomies. A Penfield No. 3 dissector, or some similar instrument, may then be inserted beneath the incised yellow ligaments in a cephalad direction, beginning at the level of the lowest laminae to be incorporated in the flap, so as to dissect the epidural fat from the spinal surfaces of the yellow ligament and laminae. This dissection is carried out from below (caudad) upward (cephalad).

Using power instruments and the finest drill blade available, one incises the laminae in a caudocephalad direction under the operating microscope, or loops, using a minimum of 3X (preferably 10X) magnification, with constant but minimal irrigation and suction. The author uses a high-speed drill, not a craniotome. The osteotomy should be made in a dorsoventral direction, proceeding along a lateral medial plane so as to provide maximum beveling, not to obtain a wedge-shaped osteotomy is but to minimize the size of the gutter and, thus, facilitate nestling it back into normal position at the time of closure. If one uses a thin cutting blade on the power instrument (less than 1 mm), bridging of the interval by bony tissue during the healing phases is greatly assisted. (Some neurosurgeons use the craniotome footplate as a guide, performing the laminotomy as one would a craniotomy. I do not suggest this technique.)

The surgeon will both feel and see the penetration through the spinal surface of the laminar cortical bone if the osteotomy is performed by using brushlike strokes in precisely the same plane. It is well to remember that individual laminae are thinner caudally where the yellow ligament is thickest and on the ventral (spinal canal) surface, whereas they are thicker cephalad where the yellow ligament is thinnest and on the dorsal surface. The laminae are osteotomized in a caudocephalad direction, but the yellow ligaments are not incised until all laminae have been osteotimized and the laminar flap is reflected. After one side of the planned flap is osteotomized in the caudocephalad direction, one returns to the contralateral, most inferior, lamina to be removed and repeats the procedure.

The laminar osteotomy is made using the high-speed drill along an imaginary line separating the pedicle from the lamina. Insertion of a curved dissector (Penefield No. 3) beneath the laminae assists the surgeon in identifying the medial surface of the pedicle and may be used to protect the epidural vessels when the laminotomy is begun. One should use the drill in brushlike strokes along the surface of the lamina in the direction of the planned line, rather than as a perforator extending through the full thickness of the lamina each time. This latter technique is dangerous; the former is safe. A fine-tipped suction tube (inserted into the laminotomy groove) and magnification allow the surgeon to see the full extent of his field. When the laminar incision is complete, the lamina may be easily moved by wedging a small dissection (Penefield No. 4) into the laminotomy groove and twisting it. This procedure is continued serially from one laminotomy to another along one side and then repeated on the other.

One then incises the interspinous ligaments between the lowest spinous process to be reflected in the flap and the highest spinous process remaining, as well as the one between the highest spinous process to be reflected and the lowest one remaining. If possible, it is desirable to make the incisions in the interspinous ligaments midway between the two appropriate spinous processes so as to facilitate closure.

In freeing the laminar flap, the yellow ligaments are cut individually on each side and at each level—preferably with a No. 15 blade mounted on a long handle—with the direction of cut being ventrodorsal so as to minimize risk of damage to the epidural structures and the dura mater. The epidural fat is stroked away from the ventral surface of the laminae with either a Penefield No. 4 or No. 3 dissection, with care being taken not to compress the dura and underlying spinal cord and/or lesion. Bridging vessels are identified, coagulated individually with bipolar cautery, and then sectioned with microscissors. As each laminar segment is freed, the laminar flap is drawn dorsally and elevated slightly cephalad so as to avoid buckling at the fulcrum, thus eliminating the risk of compressing the underlying dura and cord.

Either freshly soaked fluffy cotton or precut cottonoid patties may be placed on the dura as one reflects the laminar flap. This affords maximal protection to the underlying structures and minimizes oozing. Once the laminar flap is completely removed, fluffy cotton may be placed over the dura. The laminar flap is immediately put into normal saline, where it is left until the intraspinal operative procedure is finished.

The laminotomy flap is brought into the operative area, removing it from the moistened gauze sponge in which it was stored. If the laminar flap has been stored completely moistened, the interspinous ligaments will not have dried and shriveled. If it is stored dry, shrinkage occurs (rendering reapproximation of the laminar flap difficult or impossible).

A high-speed drill is used to perforate each of the laminae at the caudal and cranial ends of the laminar flap and the portion of the laminae that remained in the vertebral body. With the flap brought back into its anatomical position, the surgeon passes sutures through the openings made in the most caudal laminae and then ties them securely to one another, using 2-0 suture. This is done, from caudad to cephalad, at each level. These sutures are tied down individually at each level, from one side to the other. Tying down the laminar sutures one at a time, from caudal to rostral, unfolds the flap as an open occordion and brings each of the laminae to rest at its appropriate anatomical level.

Since it is not always possible to perform an osteotomy in a medial/lateral, dorsal/ventral, oblique line (which would allow the laminae to nestle into place without falling into the spinal canal), one must tie down the closing sutures snugly, so that the flap will not impinge upon the spinal canal. After the laminar flap is thus anchored into position, the interspinous ligament at the inferior and superior segments is tied to the fragments of the homonymous ligaments below and above.

The paraspinous muscle masses are then allowed to fall into their normal position by removing the self-retaining retractors. They are sewed to the respective interspinous ligaments in two layers, deep and superficial, and the facia over the paraspinous mucles is sewed to the supraspinous ligaments. This brings muscle mass, spinous processes, and interspinous ligaments into anatomical juxtaposition and prevents the laminar flap from moving or sinking into the spinal canal. The subcutaneous tissue and skin are then closed.

Postoperative Treatment and Follow-Up of Laminotomy

The postoperative treatment consists of appropriate immobilization of the patient, which is obtained through a thoracic or lumbosacral corset for the corresponding spinal segments and a "four-poster" cervical collar or "halo" for the cervical spine. Serial X-ray controls are performed on the first day after surgery and biweekly thereafter for 6 weeks. Once there is X-ray evidence of healing across the osteotomy site, no further X-ray studies are performed, and the child may resume normal activity.

Arachnoid Closure

The closure of the arachnoid is recommended in spinal cord tumor surgery and is essential for syringomyelia. It may be closed with either interrupted or continuous 7-0 sutures.

Adequate closure of the arachnoid is guaranteed at the time of opening, since at this time the surgeon has the opportunity to identify it clearly before placing guide sutures, 7-0 or 8-0, so as to tent it. If the sutures are laid at 2- or 3-mm intervals on either side of the planned line of arachnoid incision, one may make the line of incision while drawing on these guide sutures, using them for retraction sutures after the arachnoid has been opened. They may then be brought medially and tied to one another at the beginning of the arachnoid closure.

Dura Closure

The dura is closed with interrupted 4-0 sutures in the same manner as the dura over the brain, remembering that the spinal cord dura consists of only one layer and that it is, consequently, more easily frayed. If, as is so often the case, one does not get an adequate, water-tight closure, it is advisable to insert a fascial patch graft. Dural cerebral spinal fluid (CSF) leaks may compromise wound healing either by resulting in a collection of subcutaneous CSF (seroma) or by leaking through the skin incision. Both necessitate reoperation. The latter increases the risk of infection. Consequently, dural grafts should be inserted without hesitation at the slightest suggestion that the closure may not be water-tight (1).

The surgical considerations relevant to the dysraphic state and hamartomas (including the lipomeningoceles etc.) are described in a subsequent chapter: Classification and treatment of the Dysraphic State and Hamartomas.

References

1. Raimondi AJ: Pediatric Neurosurgery - Theory and art of surgical techniques. New York: Springer-Verlag, 1987.
2. Tachdjian MO, Matson DD: Orthopaedic aspects of intraspinal tumors in infants and children. J Bone Joint Surg [Am] 47:223–248, 1965.
3. Cattell HS, Clark GL Jr: Cervical kyphosis and instability following multiple laminectomies in children. J Bone Joint Surg [Am] 49:731–720, 1967.
4. Bette H, Englehardt H: Folgezustände von Laminektomien an der Halswirbelsäule. Z Orthop 85: 564–573, 1955.
5. Raimondi AJ, Gutierrez FA, Di Rocco C: Laminectomy and total reconstruction of the posterior spinal arch for spinal canal surgery in childhood. J Neurosurg 45:555–560, 1976.
6. Yasuoka S, Peterson HA, Laws ER, et al.: Pathogenesis and prophylasis of postlaminetomy deformity of the spine after multiple level laminectomy: Difference between children and adults. Neurosurgery 9:145–151, 1981.
7. Barbera J, Gonzales H, Esquerdo J, et al.: Prophylaxis of the laminectomy membrane: An experimental study in dogs. J Neurosurg 49:419–424, 1978.
8. La Rocca H, Macnab I: The laminectomy membrane. Studies on its evolution, characteristics, effects and prophylaxis in dogs. J Bone Joint Surg [Br] 56:545–50, 1974.
9. Raimondi AJ: Reflection of a laminar flap for exposure of spinal canal in children. Clin Neurosurg 25:504–511, 1978.
10. Raimondi AJ, Gutierrez FA: Reconstruction of the posterior vertebral arch laminotomy for intraspinal surgery, in Ransohoff J (ed): Modern techniques in surgery - neurosurgery. Mt Kisco, NY: Future, 1979, pp 10–11.

CHAPTER 6

Nonsurgical Diseases of the Spinal Cord Presenting as Surgical Diseases

Joan L. Venes

Although nonsurgical diseases may, on occasion, present in such a manner as to suggest a surgical lesion of the spinal cord, most will reveal themselves during a careful history-taking and physical examination.

Paralytic Syndromes

Acute Transverse Myelopathy

This is an infrequent disorder limited almost exclusively to the thoracic cord. It is characterized by rapid progression of weakness and sensory loss. Most patients exhibit a transverse sensorimotor level, but a typical Brown-Séquard's syndrome has been noted. Rarely progression may occur over several weeks, but, in general, paralysis is complete within one or two days. Fever, meningismus, and local tenderness may be present. Back and nerve root pain are an inconstant complaint.

Most cases of acute transverse myelopathy are preceded by a childhood exanthem, vaccination (e.g., rabies), infectious mononucleosis, or nonspecific viral syndrome. Weakness generally occurs four to 18 days after the onset of the associated disease.

Epidural abscess, spontaneous rupture of an arteriovenous malformation, and multiple sclerosis are the important differential diagnoses. If pain and fever are present, myelography should be done promptly to rule out epidural abscess. Hematomyelia secondary to ruptured arteriovenous malformation may also benefit from early surgical intervention. Examination of cerebrospinal fluid in acute trasverse myelitis will generally show lymphocytosis and a slight increase in protein. This is consistent with either an abscess or a hematomyelia and is nondiagnostic. If a surgical lesion is suspected, a lumbar puncture should be deferred until myelography. Treatment of transverse myelopathy is symptomatic. Steroids have been advocated and may be of some value. Complete recovery may occur over several weeks or months, although residual deficits are not uncommon. If the diagnosis of multiple sclerosis is considered, magnetic resonance imaging (MRI) can provide early information concerning remote demyelinating lesions.

Guillain-Barré Syndrome

Roughly half of the patients with Guillian-Barré have paresthesias, which may antedate the onset of weakness by hours or, less often, days. At times these paresthesias are painful and may be misinterpreted as radicular pain. Confusion with a surgical lesion most often occurs when painful paresthesias and weakness are accompanied by papilledema. Papilledema and spinal cord dysfunction can occur with either a primary intracranial lesion and drop metastases or an ependymoma of the cord with communicating hydrocephalus. Guillain-Barré syndrome is suggested by a history of antecedent viral illness and the preservation of sensation. On those rare occasions when definitive diagnosis cannot be made by history and physical examination, a computed tomography (CT) scan of the head to rule out intracranial neoplasm or a metrizamide myelogram to rule out a cord tumor is indicated. Alternatively, MRI may be used if the quality of the images is sufficiently good to show small cord lesions.

Disorders of Potassium Metabolism

This group of rare disorders presents with episodic skeletal muscle weakness. Familial (primary) hypokalemic paralysis is transmitted as an autosomal dominant gene with high penetrance. In the absence of a family history, the abrupt onset, preservation of sensation, and almost invariable eyelid lag (myotonic reflex) serve to differentiate this from a cord lesion. Although progression of muscle weakness may be rapid, the diaphragm is usually spared.

Symptoms associated or due to hypokalemia may be the presenting feature of primary hyperaldosteronism. More common in adults, the disorder is occasionally seen in children who present with episodic, increasingly severe, lower-extremity weakness and paralysis. The finding of significant hypertension and the complaint of headache should suggest hyperaldosteronism.

Hyperkalemia as a result of potassium intoxication may be accompanied by a rapidly irreversible paralysis of limb, neck, and truck muscles in which sensory deficit and loss of deep tendon reflexes have been reported. However, in the context of impaired renal function, diabetic coma, or massive hemolytic reaction, these findings are easily recognized as being due to hyperkalemia. Confusion may arise when hyperkalemia is due to severe tissue trauma in which an associated cervical spine injury is likely. A twitching response to direct percussion of the flaccid muscle should suggest the diagnosis of hyperkalemia. Electrocardiogram (ECG) is a sensitive indicator of potassium intoxication. A serum level of 7 to 10.5 mEq/ L produces a stereotyped progression of ECG changes. Initially there is an elevation of the T wave followed by a decrease in the size of the R wave and increase in the size of the S component. At very high levels there is disappearance of the P wave and obliteration of the ST segment and finally large biphasic ST complexes.

Tethered Cord Syndromes

Friedreich's Ataxia

Pes cavus, thoracic scoliosis, and hammertoe have been shown to result from tethering of the spinal cord. They are also common early findings in Friedreich's ataxia. Unsteadiness in walking and easy fatigability usually appear between 7 and 10 years of age. There may be particular difficulty with rapid turns, and the patient may complain of vertigo. The disorder is transmitted an an autosomal recessive gene without sex predilection. A family history or the finding of spinocerebellar signs such as loss of proprioceptive and vibratory sensation suggests hereditary ataxia. The cavo-varus deformity occurring with tethered cord is invariably unilateral.

Orthopedic Syndrome

James and Lassman describe a group of patients with cavovarus deformity and slight shortening of the whole lower limb. Some had sensory loss and some had abnormal reflexes. Most had no neurocutaneous stigmata and no or minimal laminar defects. In subsequent follow-up none deteriorated, and myelograms performed in some of the earlier cases were normal. They suggest myelography be reserved for patients with either progressive neurological deficit or significant laminar defect, i.e., defects greater than a simple split in the L-5 and/or S-1 laminae.

Congenital Talipes Equinovarus

The absence of neurocutaneous stigmata and normal spine X-ray findings in the infant point to congenital medial deviation of the talus as the cause. However, in those cases in which correction cannot be maintained, careful search for indications of tethering is indicated and on rare occasion MRI may be necessary. In the infant ultrasonography can be used in place of MRI and has the advantage that sedation is not required.

Bladder Dysfunction

New onset of enuresis, recurrent urinary tract infection, or failure to achieve continence by 3 years of age should prompt a urological evaluation and may require neurological and radiological investigaton to rule out tethered cord. In the presence of laminal defects or widened interpedicular distance, MRI is indicated whenever urodynamic studies suggest a neurogenic origin for bladder dysfunction. Indeed, some surgeons feel that the finding of a "neurogenic" bladder is in and of itself an indication for radiographic evaluation. It should be noted that even in the presence of significant bony abnormalities, MRI is often negative when enuresis exists as an isolated finding.

Syndrome of Spinal Cord Neoplasia

Leukemia, Hodgkin's disease, and neuroblastoma rarely call for surgical intervention if the diagnosis is known at the time of presentation. Confusion may arise when infiltration of a peripheral nerve or nerve root causes a sciatic-like picture during a remission of leukemia. In Hodgkin's disease lepto-meningeal infiltration of the cord and nerve roots is the most common form of central nervous system involvement. If symptoms progress in the face of chemotherapy and/or radiation therapy then neurosurgical intervention is indicated.

Scoliotic Syndromes

Most patients with scoliosis cannot yet be categorized and whether they suffer from any predisposing or related factors cannot be proved. Wolff's law and the Hueter-Volkmann rule are important because they underscore the dynamic nature of scoliosis. According to Wolff's law, bone is a dynamic structure that will respond to the diverse stresses and strains of daily living over time. In scoliosis persistent lateral deviation and rotation of the vertebral column lead to increased pressure on the concave side, with remodeling of cancellous bone and wedging. The Hueter-Volkmann rule states that a pressure increase on an epiphyseal growth plate will retard its growth. In scoliosis the endochondral growth plate of the vertebral facet on the concave side is affected, leading to an increase in the concavity. Thus it can be seen that once a curve begins, progression is to be expected, although rapidity of progression and eventual outcome are highly variable.

Idiopathic Scoliosis

This represents the most common form of scoliosis and referral to a neurosurgeon would be most unusual. The curve generally begins in the preadolescent period with a female sex predilection. Convexity of the curvature is always to the right, and although the curve can progress rapidly through age 16 or 17, once maturation occurs, no further progression is expected.

Infantile Idiopathic Scoliosis

This occurs in two forms. The nonprogressive form is often referred to the neurosurgeon for evaluation of plagiocepahly and ipsilateral facial hypoplasia. When plagiocephaly is associated with torticollis, care must be taken to evaluate the cervicodorsal spine. Although most curves remain stable and may resolve, those that do progress represent some of the most severe curves and early identification of progression is needed. Generally, plagiocephaly is completely resolved by 5 or 6 years of age. The syndrome of progressive infantile idiopathic scoliosis is seen in association with mental retardation and failure to thrive. These children often die from cardiorespiratory failure in the first months or years of life.

Neurofibromatosis

A very rigid deforming curve occurs in 10% of patients. Unlike the curve in idiopathic scoliosis, the curve in neurofibromatosis progresses after maturation. The finding of hemivertebrae at the apex of a sharply angled curve may often be scondary to scoliosis (Hueter-Volkmann rule) and not primary. Earlier x-ray studies often fail to show hemivertebrae prior to or in the early stages of scoliosis. This finding on earlier films eliminates consideration of diastematomyelia and can avoid the need for myelography. The angular curve is very rigid, very deforming, and very difficult to correct. The presence of an extradural tumor at the apex of the curve must be given careful consideration prior to correction. However, these are more often associated with a milder curve.

Summary

Nonsurgical disease of the cord may be divided into three categories depending on their manner of presentation - paralytic syndromes, syndromes which resemble those seen with tethering of the spinal cord, and scoliotic syndromes. It is important when considering one of these diagnoses that consideration be given to those conditions amenable to surgical correction with which they may be confused.

A fourth cagegory, spinal cord neoplasia, is included because in certain conditions early diagnosis and initiation of appropriate medical therapies can relieve symptoms and reverse neurological deficit. Laminectomy prior to radiation is associated with a risk of kyphoscoliosis and should be avoided.

Reference

1. James CCM, Lassman LP: Spinal dysraphism. An orthopaedic syndrome in children accompanying adult forms. Arch Dis Child 35:315–323, 1960.

CHAPTER 7

Infectious Diseases of the Spine in Childhood

Warwick J. Peacock

Introduction

During childhood, infectious diseases may affect the bony and ligamentous structures of the spine or the contents of the spinal canal. In developed countries the diagnosis of spinal infections may be missed because they are infrequently encountered. In underdeveloped countries, although more common, spinal infections are often seen late in the natural history of the disease, by which time permanent neurological damage or bony deformity has already occurred.

Specific pathological entities that occur are vertebral osteomyelitis of bacterial or tuberculous origin, disk space infection, epidural abscess, and abscess of the spinal cord itself. Anatomical factors are of prime importance when trying to understand the etiology, pathology, and clinical features of spinal infections and are essential when planning treatment. The vertebral column supports the trunk and prevents telescoping and protects the enclosed spinal cord; thus, bony infection with collapse may cause deformity of the spine and compression of the spinal cord. Stability and alignment of the vertebral column are maintained by the bony architecture of each vertebra, with a key role being played by the posteriorly placed articular facet joints. Infectious foci in the spine are virtually always secondary to hematogenous spread from a site of infection elsewhere in the body.

The arterial supply to the bony spine is derived from branches of the vertebral, intercostal, and lumbar arteries. These small vessels run on the anterior surface of the vertebral bodies giving off a number of minute vessels that penetrate the cortex and ramify within the cancellous bone. At each intervertebral foramen a small artery enters the spinal canal and then divides into ascending and descending branches that anastomose freely on the dorsal surface of the vertebral bodies. From this plexus two or three small branches are given off. These enter a centrally placed nutrient foramen on the posterior surface of the bone.

The vertebral venous plexus (1) can be divided into two longitudinal systems of thin-walled, richly anastomosing, valveless veins running the entire length of the spine, one within the spinal canal and the other surrounding the vertebral column. Veins drain from the marrow of the vertebral bodies through foramina into the internal vertebral plexus, which lies outside the dura extending from the base of the skull to the sacrum. It is made up of four longitudinal veins, two of them lying posterior and two anterolateral to the dura. The internal vertebral plexus communicates through the intervertebral foramina with the external vertebral plexus. The external vertebral plexus surrounds the bony and ligamentous spine as a rich network of veins lying anterior to the vertebral bodies and posterior to the lamina, where it surrounds the transverse and articular processes. Because this plexus anastomoses with the internal vertebral venous plexus and also with the vertebral, posterior intercostal, lumbar and sacral veins, a free communication exists between the veins of the pelvic viscera, the thoracoabdominal wall, the retroperitoneal space, and the posterior mediastinum. With any increase in abdominal or thoracic pressure, blood is forced into the vertebral venous system so that infected material from the thorax or abdomen is carried into the vertebral venous plexus where a secondary infective focus may be initiated.

The arterial supply to the spinal cord is derived from a single midline anterior spinal artery and two posterior spinal arteries situated immediately posteromedial to the dorsal root entry zone. The anterior spinal artery is formed by the union of two branches, one from the terminal portion of each vertebral artery. The posterior spinal artery may arise from the vertebral artery as it lies adjacent to the medulla or, more frequently, from the posterior inferior cerebellar artery. The longitudinal vessels are supplemented by radicular arteries on the anterior and posterior nerve rootlets and are derived from the vertebral, ascending cervical, posterior intercostal, and lumbar arteries. One of the anterior radicular arteries is termed the *arteria radicularis magna* (being considerably larger than the others) and is associated with one of the lower thoracic or upper lumbar anterior rootlets on the left side. The veins of the spinal cord form a tortuous plexus within the pia mater, unifying to form longitudinal channels that drain via veins on the nerve roots to the external vertebral plexus.

Spinal Epidural Abscesses

An acute spinal epidural abscess produces an emergency situation that leads to permanent paraplegia if not diagnosed and dealt with expeditiously (2).

The epidural space does not circumscribe the spinal dura completely, except below the second sacral segment (3). In the cervical, thoracic, and lumbar regions the epidural space lies mainly dorsal to the nerve roots and the dural sheath (Fig. 7.1). Anteriorly, the dura is adherent to the

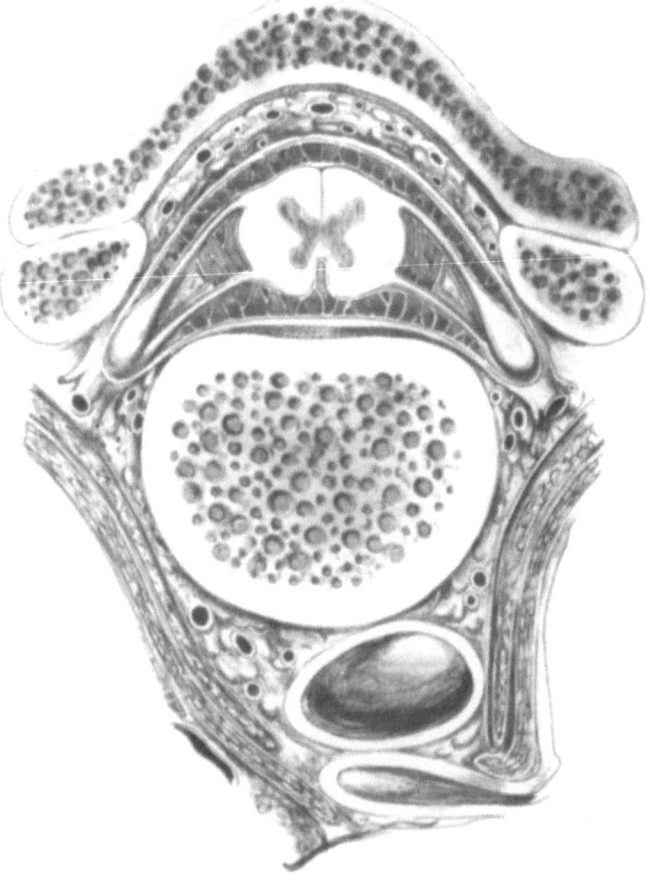

Figure 7.1. Cross-section of the spinal canal in the thoracic region showing the deep epidural space posterior to the dura filled with fat and blood vessels.

posterior longitudinal ligament with no fatty or venous intervention (3). Having left the dural sheath, the nerve roots exit from the spinal canal through the anteriorly placed intervertebral foramina, holding the dural tube against the backs of the vertebral bodies. The space between the dura and the lamina is filled with fat, loose areolar tissue and venous plexuses. It is deepest between the fourth and eighth thoracic vertebrae and from the third lumbar through the fourth sacral segments (3) (Fig. 7.2).

Although infection in the epidural space is easily transmitted along veins entering the epidural space via the intervertebral foramina from the pelvis, retroperitoneum, and posterior mediastinum (4), hematogenous spread from a distant site is the usual mode of infection, with a cutaneous furuncle being the most common source. Other primary sites of infection are otitis

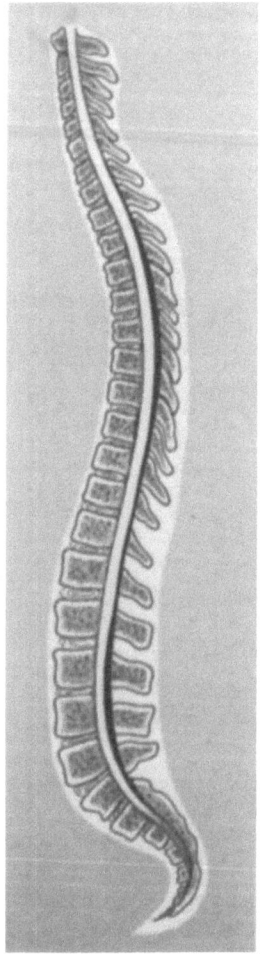

Figure 7.2. Sagittal section of the spinal column and canal showing the epidural space to be widest posteriorly in the upper thoracic and lumbar regions.

media and mastoiditis, dental abscesses, cellulitis, pyelonephritis, and pneumonia (4). Because of the frequency with which this condition is reportedly preceded by trauma (4), a predisposing factor may be an epidural hematoma that becomes infected by a coincidental bacteremia. Implantation of infection by a stab wound or lumbar puncture has been reported but is exceedingly rare (5). The most frequently isolated causative organism is *Staphylococcus aureus,* although anaerobic bacteria and *Cryptococcus* have been reported (2,4,6-12). Once established, the infected focus enlarges until there is a collection of pus deep to the laminae and ligamenta flava, lying on the dorsal surface of the dura. The pus is surrounded by thrombosed veins and granulation tissue, but because of the loose attachments and the venous plexuses, extensive longitudinal spread of suppuration may occur within the spinal canal. The infective process usually covers a number of segments, occasionally extending from the base of the skull to the sacrum, with the most common level being the midthoracic followed by the lumbosacral. Dissection into paraspinal soft tissues sometimes occurs (11).

The spinal dura provides a formidable barrier to infection, preventing the development of meningitis unless the barrier is compromised by lumbar puncture. However, the spinal cord is defenseless against inevitable compression and may also be damaged by venous or arterial thrombosis.

Clinically, spinal epidural abscess presents as a painful, febrile spinal syndrome (8). In the preparalytic phase the child complains of deep-seated backache, usually in the midthoracic region, with pain radiating around the chest wall. The pain is annoying, constant, and at times throbbing. It is made more intense by coughing, sneezing, and any movement of the spine, and is frequently associated with tenderness over the painful area (11,12). As soon as spinal cord compression occurs, weakness in the legs, with sphincter disturbance, rapidly progresses to complete and permanent paraplegia.

Examination in the preparalytic phase reveals a toxic febrile child with a stiff neck, who is exquisitely tender to percussion over the involved spinal segments. A local swelling over the spine is not uncommon in children (11), and an obvious source of infection may be found at a distant site in the skin, ears, chest, or abdomen. Spinal cord compression is manifested by finding reduced power and sensation in one or both legs and evidence of a full bladder.

In spinal epidural abscess the white blood cell count is raised and the erythrocyte sedimentation rate is elevated; a blood culture may be helpful in isolating the offending organism (8). If the patient presents in the classical way, lumbar puncture should only be performed in conjunction with myelography and then with great caution. To avoid introducing organisms into the cerebrospinal fluid repeated aspirations should be made with every 5-mm advance of the needle (8). If the spinal tenderness or local swelling is in the lumbar region, the cisternal route is preferable for myelography and cerebrospinal fluid collection.

Spinal X-ray studies are helpful in excluding other causes of low backache such as disk space infection, which can simulate epidural abscesses. X-ray evidence of osteomyelitis is rarely present (2), but the absence of radiological abnormalities does not exclude the diagnosis. Myelography will show either an extradural mass or a complete extradural block. Using the clinical and myelographic information, the extent of the epidural abscess may often be determined prior to surgery. Computerized tomography (CT) with metrizamide (Fig. 7.3) or magnetic resonance imaging (MRI) have superseded standard myelography.

The differential diagnosis includes osteomyelitis of the spine, both bacterial and tuberculous, the Guillain-Barré syndrome, acute transverse myelopathy, poliomyelitis, disk space infection, spontaneous spinal epi-

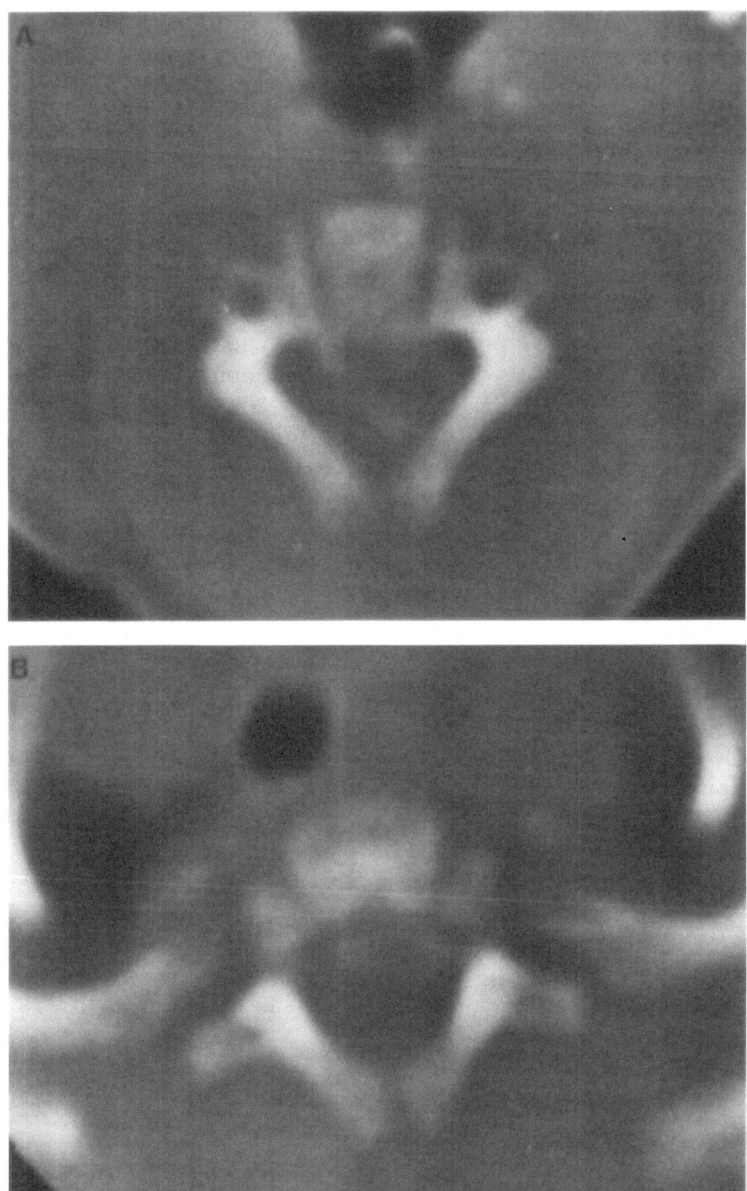

Figure 7.3. Epidural abscess. This CT metrizamide study of the cervical (**A**) and upper thoracic spines (**B**) shows an anterolateral displacement of the dural sac and spinal cord by a posteriorly situated epidural abscess.

dural hematoma (which is exceedingly rare), and extradural tumors such as neuroblastoma and epidural sarcoma (4). Tuberculosis of the vertebral column is a slowly developing disease associated with other evidence of tuberculosis and characteristic radiological changes. Pyogenic spinal osteitis tends to run a subacute or chronic course, usually being seen in elderly diabetic patients or in patients who have had recent urinary tract infection or manipulation, or are known intravenous substance abusers. The Guillain-Barré syndrome is painless, tending to produce a flaccid weakness with hyporeflexia in all four limbs. With acute transverse myelopathy there is usually no back pain, the course is rapid, and the paralysis is often preceded by a mild illness. Poliomyelitis should not be considered if there is localized back pain, sensory deficit, bladder involvement, or symmetrical motor loss. Disk space infection may mimic acute spinal epidural abscess precisely, especially in the younger child where, owing to pain precipitated by movement, assessment of motor function may be confusing.

Treatment of acute spinal epidural abscess is emergency laminectomy and decompression of the spinal canal by drainage of pus. It is not necessary to remove laminae over the entire extent of the abscess, as a two- or three-level laminectomy usually suffices (8). Catheter irrigation of involved but unexposed parts of the abscess facilitates drainage at the time of surgery. Because the responsible organism is probably *Staphylococcus aureus,* a semisynthetic penicillinase-resistant penicillin preparation should be given intravenously until the bacterial sensitivity results are available. If bladder control is compromised, an indwelling urinary catheter or intermittent catheterization should be used.

The prognosis is entirely related to preoperative neurological status. If the spinal canal is decompressed in the preparalytic phase, the patient should make a complete recovery. When mild motor weakness has been present for less than 36 hours, a good recovery is still possible; but once the stage of complete paraplegia has been reached, recovery is most unlikely (11).

Pyogenic Spondylitis

Hematogenous osteomyelitis of the long bones is common in children, whereas vertebral osteomyelitis in this age group is distinctly rare (13). In a reported series of pyogenic spondylitis, more than 80% of cases were adults (14). Although this condition is infrequently seen in children, it is important because of the difficulty of diagnosis and the serious consequences of delayed treatment.

Although *Staphylococcus aureus* is the most common causative organism, gram-negative rods, including *Escherichia coli, Pseudomonas aeruginosa, Klebsiella,* and *Salmonella* have been implicated (14,15). The infection reaches the vertebral body via the bloodstream but may extend to involve the bony vertebral arch. The thoracic or lumbar vertebrae are most frequently affected. The abscess in the vertebral body may rupture under the anterior longitudinal ligament to produce a paraspinal soft-tissue abscess. If the abscess extends posteriorly, pus collects in the epidural space, but this is uncommon. With progressive destruction bony collapse and kyphos formation occurs but if the sepsis is less destructive, bony sclerosis develops with spontaneous arthrodesis.

In pyogenic spondylitis of infancy the early clinical features are often obscure, but include irritability, fever, failure to thrive, diarrhea, and pain associated with movement. Absence of localizing findings can make the early diagnosis difficult unless this condition is borne in mind. In older children and adolescents, predisposing factors such as substance abuse, instrumentation of the urinary tract, or chronic hemodialysis are sometimes present (16). Back pain, the usual presenting complaint, is more often gradual than abrupt in onset and is frequently accompanied by radicular pain. In atypical cases back pain may be entirely absent, with symptoms and signs referable only to the abdomen (16). Fever is a usual, but not constant, accompaniment, and there is local tenderness and pain on axial compression. A local or remote fluctuant mass may be found.

The white blood cell count is not always raised, while the erythrocyte sedimentation rate is invariably elevated; blood culture is helpful in isolating the organisms (16). X-ray studies are of little assistance in the early stages, but within 4 to 6 weeks a paravertebral shadow may be the first sign of spinal disease (13). A few weeks later, focal destructive changes adjacent to the cartilaginous end plate can be detected and eventually lytic destruction in the central region of the body is seen. This may progress to collapse and kyphotic deformity (Fig. 7.4, 7.5). Early in the disease process isotope bone scans may be the only helpful investigation, but later tomography and CT scanning are able to detect disturbances of bony integrity. Needle or open biopsy of an associated abscess may be essential to isolate the offending organism.

The key to successful management is recognition because the condition is uncommon and repeatedly omitted from the differential diagnosis. Essential to treatment are rest, supportive measures, antibiotics, and, when necessary, surgery. Accurate antibiotic therapy is dependent on the sensitivity report, but until this is available, a cephalosporin and an aminoglycoside are good choices; serial erythrocyte sedimentation rates can be used to monitor the effectiveness of therapy. Operative treatment is required if there has been abscess formation, if a draining sinus has developed, or if conservative measures have failed to control the bony sepsis. An anterior approach allows debridement, with removal of septic deposits and sequestra. If there is evidence of spinal cord involvement, the posterior longitudinal ligament should be removed and the dura exposed. A bone graft made of struts of pelvis or a fibular strut prevents deformity. Fusion occurs rapidly.

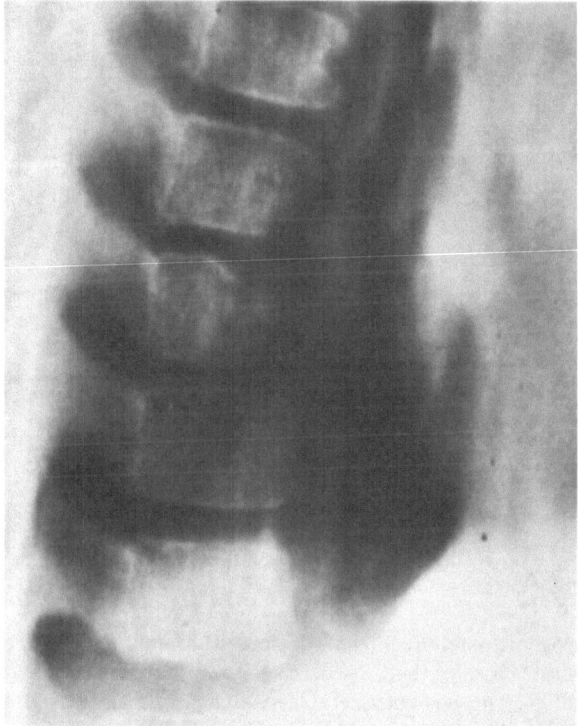

Figure 7.4. Pyogenic osteomyelitis of the spine. Lateral radiograph of the thoracic spine shows erosion and compression of the T-8 vertebral body with narrowing of the T8-9 disk space.

Disk Space Infections in Children

Although an argument has been put forward that discitis in childhood is not an infective condition (17), there are many authors who believe that bacterial infection is present in the disk space (18–20). Intervertebral disk space infections affect children in a distinctive clinical manner. They occur most commonly between the ages of 4 and 11, but cases in which the patients were under 2 years of age have been encountered (20). There has often been a preceding febrile illness or history of trauma before the characteristic clinical syndrome starts, and the patient either complains of low back pain or exhibits physical findings suggestive of back pain. The pain that is aggravated by activity is often present at night, and there is a progression from refusal to stand or walk to refusal to sit. Fever rarely exceeds 102°F, but some patients remain afebrile.

Paraspinal muscle spasm is often present and spinous process tenderness can be elicited. In very young children it may be extremely difficult to differentiate between hip pathology and discitis because the child refuses

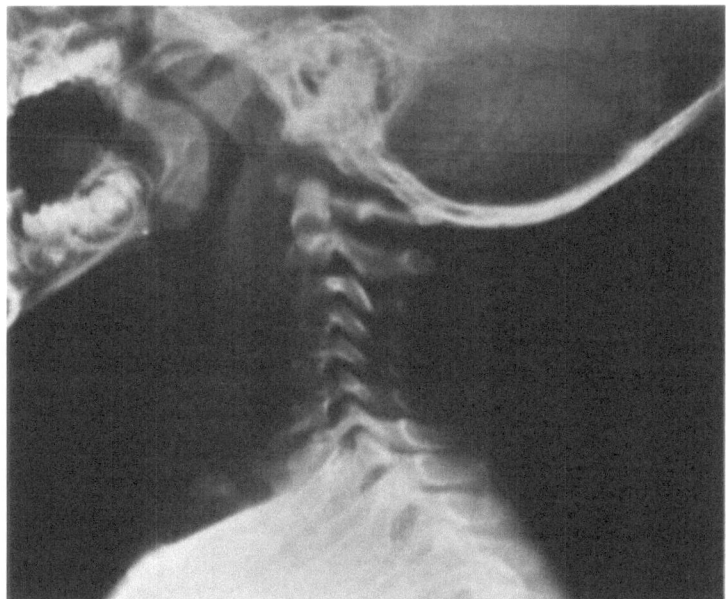

Figure 7.5. Pyogenic osteomyelitis of the spine. Lateral radiograph of the cervical spine demonstrates loss of the C3-4 disk space and erosion of the anterior aspect of the body of C-4. There is considerable swelling of the prevertebral soft tissues, and C-2 is displaced anteriorly relative to C-3.

to actively move one or both lower limbs and passive movement appears to produce intense pain. Spinal disease may also produce hip pain, but the two causes of pain can usually be differentiated clinically. In hip disease percussion over the greater trochanter and palpation over the posterior aspect of the hip produces pain and extension of the thigh is restricted (20). True weakness may be present, but tendon reflexes are rarely absent (21).

An elevated erythrocyte sedimentation rate is the most significant and consistent laboratory finding (18,20). The white blood cell count is often, but not always, mildly elevated and is rarely more than 15,000/μL (20). Radiographic changes are not usually present for 2 to 4 weeks after the onset of the illness. The earliest change is disk-space narrowing below the ninth thoracic vertebra, with the majority occurring in the lumbar region (Fig. 7.6). The bony margin adjacent to the affected disk space becomes demineralized and irregular, with evidence of bony destruction. The narrowing persists for 4 to 12 weeks while the bony margins become sclerotic. In most cases the intervertebral space widens over 2 to 8 months (18). If straight X-ray studies are not helpful in the early stages, tomography may show the early changes, and an isotope bone scan can prove the pathology is localized to the vertebral column (Fig. 7.7). Repeated spinal

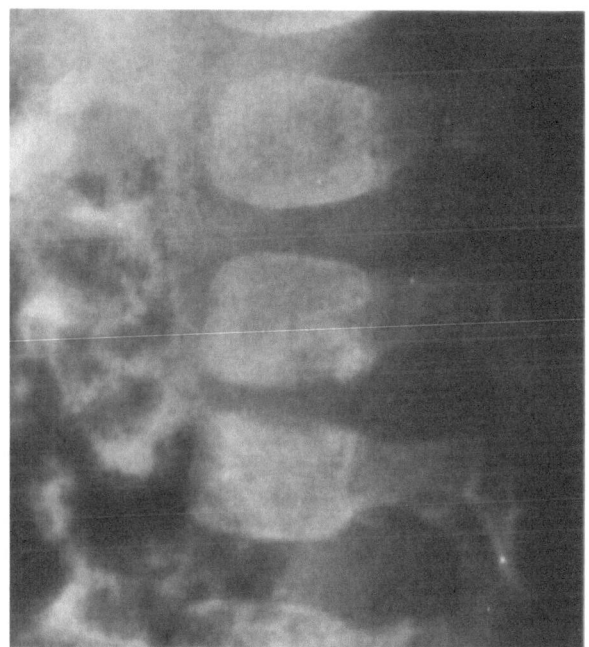

Figure 7.6. Discitis. Lateral radiograph of a 2½-year-old girl with the clinical features of discitis. The L2-3 disk space is narrowed, and there is some erosion of the inferior aspect of the body of L-2.

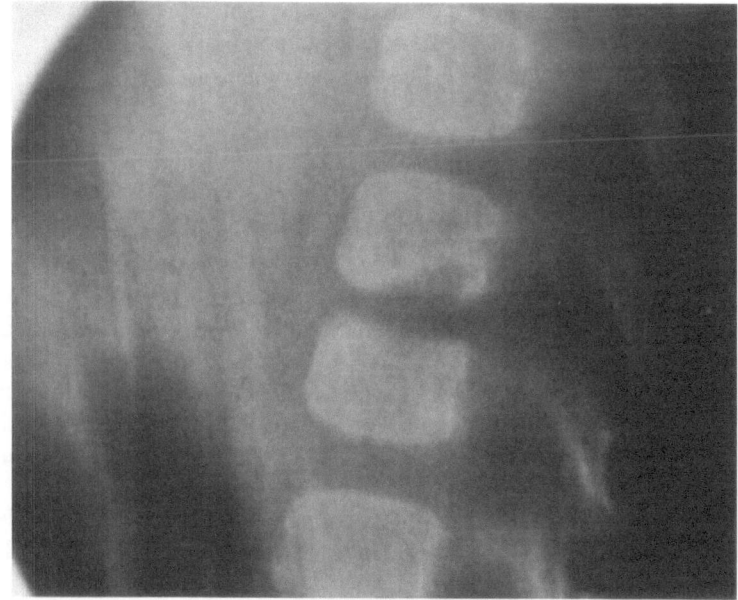

Figure 7.7. Discitis. Midsagittal tomograph demonstrates more clearly the erosion of the body of L-2.

X-ray studies are often necessary before changes can be detected. Disk space biopsy or aspiration is not advised in the typical case, as a pathogenic organism is discovered in less than one third of cases. *Staphylococcus aureus* has been the most commonly isolated organism, but gram-negative bacilli such as *Escherichia coli* or *Proteus mirabilis* have been isolated in children with preceding urinary tract infections (18).

Alexander (17) queried the infectious basis of juvenile spondyloarthritis. He proposed that although occasional cases of discitis are due to infection, the vast majority are due to partial dislocation of the epiphysis during a flexion injury. He states that deep radial notching develops at about 7 years of age on the upper and lower surfaces of thoracic and lumbar vertebral bodies and protects the epiphyseal plates from tangential sheer stresses. This could explain why the condition occurs infrequently beyond the age of 7 years.

The majority of writers, however, (18–20), believe that most cases of discitis are due to infection and treat the patients with antibiotics, monitoring progress with serial erythrocyte sedimentation rate assessments. These authors have reported prompt resolution and pain relief following antibiotic administration (18–20).

Persistence, patience, and a high index of suspicion are needed to make this diagnosis. When a febrile but not acutely ill child has intense back pain and refuses to walk or sit, and if the sedimentation rate is raised, although the white blood cell count may not be, this condition should be considered even if the results of straight spinal radiographs are normal. By repeating x-ray studies and by doing an isotope bone scan, a diagnosis will eventually be reached. With correct management the outlook is excellent (21).

Spinal Cord Abscess

This is an extremely uncommon but important condition, as it has become potentially curable since the advent of antibiotics combined with appropriate surgery (22). A spinal cord abscess is usually produced by blood-spread infection from a primary site such as endocarditis, bronchiectasis, or middle-ear infection, with *Staphylococcus* and *Streptococcus* being the organisms most frequently isolated (23). Direct implantation by lumbar puncture or stab wound (23) and spread from a dermal sinus (24) have been reported; in one fourth of the cases no primary site of infection can be found (25,26).

Multiple abscesses are occasionally found, with the thoracic cord being the most common site followed by the cervical and lumbar segments. Early on there is a purulent myelitis in which central softening and necrosis occur with capsule formation (25).

Clinically, the patient has features of infection, back or neck pain, and progressive neurological deficit. If the course is acute with full evolution within a few days, the prognosis is poor and the mortality rate approaches 90% (25). When the clinical course is less rapid and the features are similar to those of an intramedullary tumor, the outcome is more hopeful. Plain X-ray studies are rarely helpful, whereas myelography will show widening of the cord with complete obstruction to the flow of contrast medium. The cerebrospinal fluid shows features of meningitis but is usually sterile. The MRI is the investigation of choice.

Treatment (27) consists of antibiotic administration with decompressive laminectomy and drainage via a midline myelotomy. As the organisms are usually penicillinase-resistant, methicillin and chloramphenicol are appropriate until the aerobic and anaerobic cultures are available. Dexamethasone is probably indicated to reduce cord swelling.

Tuberculous Spondylitis (Pott's Disease)

Although this ancient disease is known to have produced vast amounts of human suffering from the time of the early Egyptians, it has only been during the last 30 years that it has been brought under control and then only in the technologically advanced nations of the world. In the underdeveloped countries it continues to devastate large numbers of patients, especially children.

Tuberculosis of the spine is probably always secondary to an active primary focus elsewhere in the body, although this is often not apparent. The tubercle bacillus that causes skeletal tuberculosis may be of the human or bovine variety. In the early years of this century, more than half the reported cases were infected with the bovine bacillus (28), but since measures were introduced to ensure a clean supply of milk, today only the human bacillus is found to be responsible (29). The primary focus lies in the lungs and spread is via the bloodstream to the spine. The most common part of the vertebral column affected is the lower thoracic region, with the lumbar and cervical spine less commonly involved (30). In 5% to 10% of cases there are double lesions with intervening normal vertebrae.

The disease begins as an infection of two adjacent vertebral bodies where, owing to tuberculous endarteritis, the marrow becomes devitalized and caseous. Because of superimposed weight, the vertebral bodies eventually collapse, producing a kyphotic spinal deformity (30). If the disease process spreads to adjacent vertebrae, the magnitude of the deformity is increased, and in children, three or four vertebral bodies are frequently affected. With bony collapse, tuberculous debris collects under the anterior longitudinal ligament and may track downward as a cold abscess. With cervical disease a retropharyngeal abscess results, whereas in the lower thoracic or lumbar region a cold abscess may be produced that points in the groin or in Petit's lumbar triangle. If the abscess tracks posteriorly, debris collects in the spinal canal where the spinal cord may be compressed producing an early paraplegia. Late paraplegia results from peridural fibrosis and endarteritis of the feeding vessels of the spinal cord; it is probably also related to traction and attrition of the cord due to the internal gibbus.

The patient has a history of chronic illness and recent onset of spinal pain, which may be associated with radicular pain. Children frequently present because they stop walking (not due to leg weakness) or the mother notices the gibbus. Neurological signs due to spinal cord involvement are present in up to one third of patients (31). There is usually local tenderness and sometimes swelling, with paraspinal muscle spasm and restricted movement; spinal deformity in the form of a gibbus or kyphos is found if vertebral collapse has occurred (Fig. 7.8). Soft-tissue swellings due to cold abscess formation should be looked for, and if the disease is advanced, discharging sinuses may be present. When the spinal cord is affected, weakness in the legs and sensory loss can be detected. Eventually the sphincters become involved. Bailey et al. (32) reported their findings with 100 children suffering from tuberculous spondylitis. A total of 76 children

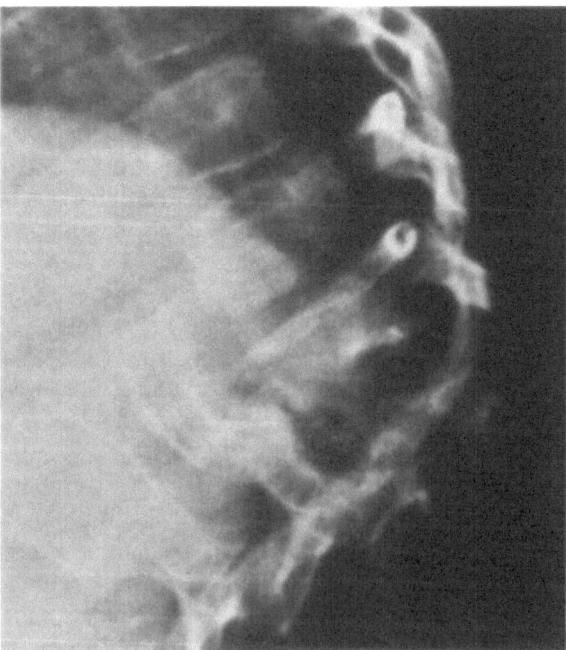

Figure 7.8. Tuberculous osteitis of the spine. Lateral radiograph of the spine demonstrates a short gibbus deformity at the thoracolumbar junction with severe collapse and compression of two vertebral bodies and erosion of the next most caudal vertebral body.

were under 5 years of age, and the thoracic location was the most common. Seventy-four patients showed a kyphos and 34 a scoliosis. On average, three vertebrae were involved, and only two were collapsed. On admission, 43 children were paraplegic, but only seven failed to recover completely. Twenty-seven children had active pulmonary tuberculosis.

The cornerstone of diagnosis is the identification of tubercle bacilli in the lesion which is best achieved by needle biopsy under fluoroscopic control. No other study, however helpful, is conclusive, for even the isolation of acid-fast bacilli from the sputum or urine does not prove that the spinal lesion is tuberculous. Pyogenic spondylitis due to *Staphylococci,* gram-negative bacteria, or associated with typhoid or brucellosis may mimic spinal tuberculosis. There is, however, less bone destruction and, consequently, less deformity than with tuberculosis. Unlike what is seen with tuberculosis, the vertebral margins show evidence of bone reaction manifested on X-ray by bone sclerosis. An eosinophilic granuloma can cause collapse of a vertebral body, closely resembling tuberculous vertebral destruction, but the disk space remains intact. Anteroposterior and lateral spinal X-ray studies in Pott's disease typically show involvement of the body, with sparing of the arch structures. The lateral view shows evidence of disease before the anteroposterior view (Fig. 7.9). Initially, there is disk narrowing, and then the body becomes wedge-shaped. In the active stage the bone loses density. Progressive destruction of bone occurs with very little evidence of reactive change; ultimately, one or more vertebral bodies collapse, producing a gibbus or kyphos. The anteroposterior view will show a paravertebral shadow in more than half the cases, but in a larger number a paravertebral abscess will be found at surgery. The radiological hallmark of tuberculous spondylitis is anterior collapse or wedging of two adjacent vertebrae, with loss of disk space on the X-ray film (although at surgery the disk is often still present). With the bony softening, the disk has intruded into the vertebral bodies. An MRI scan shows the disk space, bony pathology, and any narrowing of the spinal canal (Fig. 7.10).

Management

Primary therapy for tuberculous spondylitis is chemical, based ideally on bacteriologic identification and sensitivity studies. In the early days of antituberculous therapy, isoniazid, aminosalicylic acid, and streptomycin were standard. The introduction of newer drugs, such as rifampin, ethambutol, and others, has made control much easier.

The goals of management are, first, bacteriologic control and, second, a stable spine with minimal deformity. Although chemotherapeutic agents do gain access into the caseous lesion, surgery may be required if there has been much bony destruction, if large abscesses have collected, or if the spinal cord is in danger. The decision is usually made in individual cases according to the response to conservative treatment.

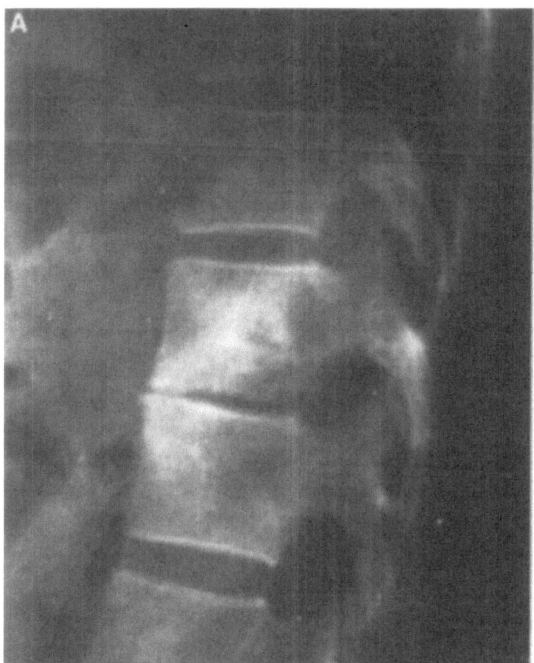

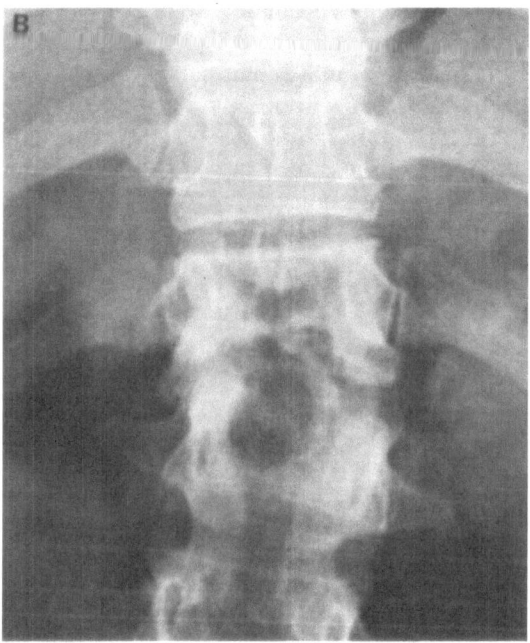

Figure 7.9. Tuberculous osteitis of the spine. Anteroposterior (**A**) and lateral (**B**) radiographs of the thoracolumbar region show marked thinning of the T12-L1 disk space with erosion and sclerosis of the two adjacent vertebral bodies.

Figure 7.10. Tuberculous osteitis of the spine. Midsagittal
MRI scan using a T-1 weighted
technique shows loss of detail at
the T12-L1 disk space, slight
decrease in signal intensity of
the two involved vertebral bodies, and encroachment upon the
spinal canal.

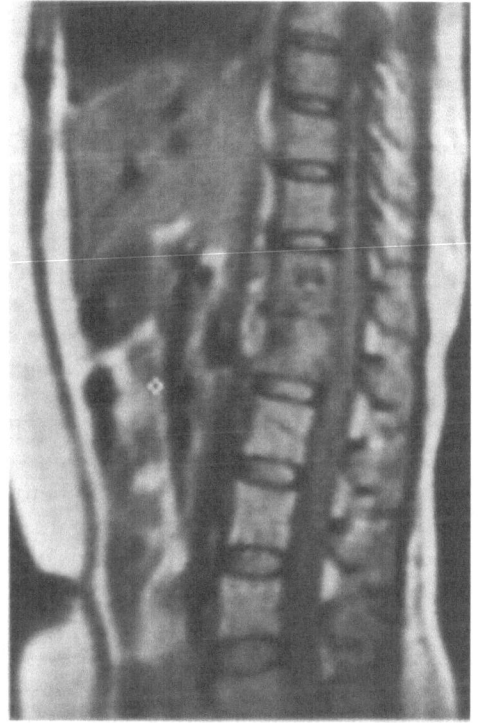

In treating tuberculous spondylitis the three elements of this condition
must be borne in mind: the infectious process, the bony destruction plus
deformity, and the neurological involvement. If the infection is inade-
quately treated, deformity and paralysis may result; if the deformity is
neglected, it may also lead to paralysis and, in addition, cause restrictive
pulmonary disease and heart failure.

Management of spinal tuberculosis in different centers varies from am-
bulant chemotherapy alone to radical anterior debridement and grafting
(33). The decision whether to operate or not depends on the site and extent
of vertebral involvement, severity of the kyphos, presence and size of
paravertebral abscesses, neurological involvement, and response to
chemotherapy. Local factors, such as the availability of facilities for specialized surgical procedures, must obviously be taken into account. Multiple-level vertebral involvement in the thoracic spine is likely to cause
either early- or late-onset paraplegia. It tends also to produce a kyphos
of sufficient severity to cause respiratory embarrassment. Early radical
surgery with an anterior supporting bone graft is therefore justified. The
greater the number of vertebral bodies that are destroyed, the more urgent
is the need for supporting the spine anteriorly by bone strut grafting to
prevent further collapses. Rib or iliac crest grafts frequently fracture, es-

pecially when they span a large gap, whereas a fibular graft forms an immediate strong support, although its incorporation takes longer. Posterior spinal fusion alone, even when there is minimal deformity, and especially if three or more vertebrae are involved, may not prevent progression of the kyphosis. Involvement of a single level with minimal deformity and no neurological deficit may not require surgery; it can be treated effectively with chemotherapy alone, although careful follow-up is important.

Spinal deformity is a cause of serious disability in spinal tuberculosis. A major thoracic kyphyosis produces restrictive pulmonary disease, which eventually leads to pulmonary hypertension and right-sided heart failure. At best, the cosmetic aspect of a "hunchback" deformity is an unwanted complication. Late-onset paraplegia results from bony impingement from the tuberculous kyphosis at the front of the cord, but the spinal cord shows marked resilience in some cases with severe deformities. During the healing phase, the consolidating mass of tuberculous pus encircling the dura may produce a fibrous stricture leading to late-onset paraplegia. With a condition as devastating as tuberculosis of the spine, cosmetic considerations are often neglected until the infection is controlled; only then is the psychological impact on the patient appreciated. However, it is illogical not to prevent the severe deformities associated with this disease. This can only be done by an early anterior strut bone graft in cases of multiple-level involvement or severe spinal curvature.

References

1. Batson OV: The function of the vertebral veins and their role in the spread of metastases. Ann Surg 112:138–149, 1940.
2. Enberg RN, Kaplan RJ: Spinal epidural abscess in children. Clin Pediatr 13:247–253, 1974.
3. Dandy WE: Abscesses and inflammatory tumors in the spinal epidural space. Arch Surg 13:477–494, 1926.
4. Fischer EG, Greene CS, Winston KR: Spinal epidural abscess in children. Neurosurgery 9:257–260, 1981.
5. Peacock WJ, Shrosbree RD, Key AG: A review of 450 stabwounds of the spinal cord. S Afr Med J 51:961–964, 1977.
6. Heusner AP: Nontuberculous spinal epidural infections. N Engl J Med 239:48–53, 1948.
7. Bergman I, Wald E, Meyer JDS, et al.: Epidural abscess and vertebral osteomyelitis following serial lumbar punctures. Pediatrics 72:476–480, 1983.
8. deVilliers JC, Cluver PF deV: Spinal epidural abscess in children. S Afr J Surg 16:149–155, 1978.
9. Gasul BM, Jaffe RH: Acute spinal epidural abscess - a clinical entity. Arch Pediatr 52:361–390, 1935.
10. Baker CJ: Primary spinal epidural abscess. Am J Dis Child 121:337–339, 1971.
11. Hulme A, Dott NM: Spinal epidural abscess. Br Med J 1:64–68, 1954.
12. Browden J, Meyers R: Pyogenic infections of the spinal epidural space. Surgery 10:296–308, 1941.

13. Kulowski J: Pyogenic osteomyelitis of the spine. J Bone Joint Surg 18:343–364, 1936.
14. Wiley AM, Trueta J: The vascular anatomy of the spine and its relationship to pyogenic vertebral osteomyelitis. J Bone Joint Surg 41B:796–809, 1959.
15. Griffiths HED, Jones DM: Pyogenic infection of the spine. J Bone Joint Surg 53B:383–391, 1971.
16. Bolivar R, Kohl S, Pickering L: Vertebral osteomyelitis in children: report of four cases. Pediatrics 62:549–553, 1978.
17. Alexander CJ: The aetiology of juvenile spondyloarthritis (discitis). Clin Radiol 21:148–187, 1970.
18. Milone FP, Bianco AJ, Ivins JC: Infections of the intervertebral disk in children. JAMA 181:1029–1033, 1962.
19. Rubin CR, Jacobs BG, Cooper PR et al.: Disc space infections in children. Childs Brain 3:180–190, 1977.
20. Lascari AD, Graham MH, MacQueen JC: Intervertebral disk infection in children. J Pediatr 70:751–757, 1967.
21. Matson DD: Neurosurgery of infancy and childhood, 2 ed. Springfield Ill: Charles C Thomas Publisher, 1969, p 737.
22. Rifaat M, El Shafei I, Samra K, et al.: Intramedullary spinal abscess following spinal puncture. J Neurosurg 38:366–367, 1973.
23. Wright RL: Intramedullary spinal cord abscess. J Neurosurg 23:208–210, 1965.
24. Gindi SE, Fairburn B: Intramedullary spinal abscess as a complication of a congenital dermal sinus. J Neurosurg 30:494–497, 1969.
25. Menezes AH, Graf CJ, Pevret G: Spinal cord abscess: a review. Surg Neurol 8:461–467, 1977.
26. Artz PK: Abscess within the spinal cord; review of literature and report of three cases. 51:533–543, 1944.
27. Menezes AH, Van Gilder JC: Spinal cord abscess, in Wilkins RH, Rengachary SS (eds): Neurosurgery. New York: McGraw-Hill, 1985, pp 1969–1979.
28. Bick EM: Source book of orthopedics. New York: Hafner, 1948, pp 5–6.
29. Campos OP: Bone and joint tuberculosis and its treatment. J Bone Joint Surg 37B:937–966, 1955.
30. Hodgson AR: Tuberculosis of the spine, in Ruge D, Wiltse LL (eds): Spinal disorders. Philadelphia; Lea & Febiger, 1977, pp 102–114.
31. Hodgson AR, Stock FE: Anterior spine fusion for the treatment of tuberculosis of the spine. J Bone Joint Surg 42B:295–310, 1960.
32. Bailey HL, Gabriel M, Hodgson AR, et al.: Tuberculosis of the spine in children. J Bone Joint Surg 54B:1633–1657, 1972.
33. Medical Research Working Party on Tuberculosis of the Spine: Five year assessment of controlled trials of ambulatory treatment debridement and anterior spinal fusion in the management of tuberculosis of the spine. Studies in Bulawago (Zimbabwe) and in Hong Kong. J Bone Surg 60B:163–177, 1978.

CHAPTER 8

Parasitosis of the Spine

Adelola Adeloye

Schistosomiasis of the Spinal Cord

This trematode worm infestation is also called bilharziasis, after Bilharz, who in 1851 first described the parasite (1). It is estimated that about 200 million people, including children, are infested with this parasite in different parts of the world (2). There are three species of the worm, namely *Schistosoma haematobium, Schistosoma mansoni,* and *Schistosoma japonicum.* The species *S. haematobium,* with its terminal-spined eggs, and *S. mansoni,* with its lateral-spined eggs, are prevalent in northern parts of Egypt, in the Rift Valley area, the great lakes of East and Central Africa, the Near East, the West Coast of Africa, and the North Coast of South America, including Brazil. *Schistosoma japonicum,* with oval eggs and a rudimentary lateral spine or knob, is common in the Far East (3).

Incidence

The occurrence of schistosomiasis of the spinal cord is probably higher than what has been documented. The 43 cases of the disease collected by Norfray et al. (4) consisted of 24 from Africa, 11 from South America (Brazil, 9; Venezuela, 2), and 8 from Puerto Rico. The 24 African cases comprised 10 from South Africa, 6 from Egypt, 3 from Sudan, 2 each from Nigeria and Uganda, and one from Morocco.

Males are predominantly more affected than females, and about 75% of the patients are aged between 10 and 35 years.

Pathology

Distribution of the Parasites

Schistosoma haematobium mainly affects the spinal cord, whereas *S. mansoni* affects the brain and cord, more often the latter. *Schistosoma japonicum* predominantly affects the brain; it rarely invades the spinal cord. Levy et al. (5) described the number of cases and the distribution of the parasite in the central nervous system as follows: *S. mansoni:* cord, 32; brain, 16. *S. haematobium:* cord, 13; brain, 5. *S. japonicum:* cord, 2; brain, 110.

The predominance of *S. mansoni* as a cause of spinal cord involvement has also been reported by Herskowitz (6) and Luyendijk and by Lindeman (3) who found that in a series of 26 cases, *S. mansoni* was involved in 16 cases, *S. haematobium* in nine, and *S. japonicum* in only one instance. However, it appears that in a particular locality, one species tends to predominate; the two cases reported from Ibadan, Nigeria, were due to *S. haematobium* (7,8), and the three cases encountered in Kenya were associated with *S. mansoni* (2,9).

Mode of Cord Invasion

Involvement of the brain and spinal cord by the parasite is usually by the ova; how the adult worm and its ova reach the central nervous system is uncertain. Mechanical and immunological pathways have been suggested to explain parasitic invasion of the brain and spinal cord. The mechanical pathways are summarized as follows:

1. Embolization of ova is said to occur through collaterals to the paravertebral valveless venous plexus of Batson (10) and its intracranial connection. This pathway is similar to that taken by metastases from prostatic carcinoma to reach the lumbar vertebrae.
2. Arterial embolization of aberrant worms in the pulmonary vascular bed has also been suggested (11). The large anterior radicular artery entering the spinal canal near the lower end of the dorsal spine would explain why the favorite site of spinal lesions in schistosomiasis is the conus medullaris.
3. Migration of the worms in the venous pathways close to the spine and the deposition of their ova in the same area may occur. Marciel et al. (12) suggested that obstruction of an emissary vein of the spinal plexus by a female worm loaded with eggs may lead to the parasite being sucked into the intramedullary venous plexus. This has been offered to explain the dural and extradural lesions of spinal bilharziasis.

As for the *immunological* pathways, Cohen et al. (13) attributed the development of bilharzial myelitis to the presence of circulating immunocomplexes.

Types of Spinal Cord Lesion

In the early stage of invasion of the cord by the parasite, there may be no pathological changes; Budzilovich et al. (14) demonstrated ova in the spinal cord without any inflammatory reaction. Later, the following lesions appear.

Transverse Myelitis

In this lesion, destruction, vacuolation, and atrophy of the cord occur with little reaction around the ova (15–20). The lesion tends to develop soon after exposure to bilharzia in the nonimmune subject, but much later after infection in the immunized (21).

In this variety of the disease, many small granulomata occur throughout the spinal cord. The lesions remain close together, each surrounding one or more ova. When there are many necrotic areas, permanent cord damage may occur (22).

Granulomatous Lesion

Here, a granuloma forms as a result of intense gliotic and fibrotic reaction to the ova. The granuloma may be tiny and diffuse, causing no cord damage (7,23). When it is large and solitary, the granuloma may cause neurological damage by direct pressure and cord invasion (24).

Radicular Lesion

In this type, numerous granulomata form in the spinal roots instead of in the cord (25). The distinct existence of a radicular lesion has been questioned by some authorities in the belief that the myelitic and granulomatous disease may each have a radicular component (26).

What type of lesion a patient develops appears to be dictated by the intensity of allergic response to the presence of the parasite. When tissue reaction is intense, the granulomatous lesion is produced; if the reaction is minimal, transverse myelitis develops. For unknown reasons, the granulomatous lesion occurs almost entirely in males (27).

Clinical Features

The patient with spinal cord bilharziasis is very often a boy or a juvenile aged between 10 and 20 years. No age group, however, is exempt. Dar and Zimmerman (2) in Nairobi, Kenya, reported transverse myelitis due to *S. mansoni* in a 14-month-old Kenyan male infant; the ages of the 43 patients described by Norfray et al. (4) ranged from 8 to 73 years.

All patients had a history of residing in or traveling through areas where schistosomiasis is endemic. The initial complaint in spinal cord disease is pain in the low back, the girdle, or the sciatic region. This is soon followed by *sphincter disturbances* manifested mainly as incontinence of urine. Then, *weakness* appears in the legs, beginning in one leg and involving the other leg shortly afterward. The weakness rapidly progresses so that paraplegia is established in the course of a few weeks.

Diagnosis

Spinal cord bilharziasis should be suspected under the following circumstances:

1. Characteristic symptoms and signs.
2. In a patient from an area of the world where schistosomiasis is rife.
3. History of recent exposure to the infestation. It should be noted that in about 60% of cases, there may be no evidence of schistosomiasis outside the spinal cord.
4. Leucocytosis with eosinophilia in the peripheral blood and the cerebrospinal fluid. This is a common finding, occurring in more than 50% of cases (28,29). The eosinophilia often falls with antibilharzial drugs.
5. Recovery of ova from urine or the stool.
6. Positive bilharzial skin test, which is obtained in 50% of cases.
7. A strongly positive precipitin and circumoral reaction to cerebrospinal fluid, which is specific for spinal cord disease. The precipitin test is 90% positive in early stages of the disease, but falls to 50% in the chronic stages (6,29).
8. With the exception of nos 4 and 7 above, lumbar puncture findings are more normal than abnormal.

Radiological Features

Plain radiograms of the spine are usually normal. Myelography is helpful in granulomatous disease in which the following characteristic features occur.

1. Myelographic block of a size equal to the length of a vertebral body and located opposite the bodies of D-12 and L-1. This is the most common level of involvement (30).
2. Irregular trifid edges at the upper end of the granuloma. El-Banhawy's (26) "three-finger appearance" is pathognomonic of the disease (Fig. 8.1).
3. Abrupt intramedullary swelling, unlike other intramedullary tumors, which tend to taper gradually at one end.
4. The picture of extradural, subdural, or complete spinal blockage may also be produced on myelography.

Treatment

Bilharzial myelitis is treated by antibilharzial drugs alone, usually with complete clinical and radiological recovery (31). Drug treatment alone is also adequate in early granulomatous disease.

   Treatment of moderate to large *bilharzial granuloma*, the type that commonly confronts the surgeon, is not as easy. The rapid course of the

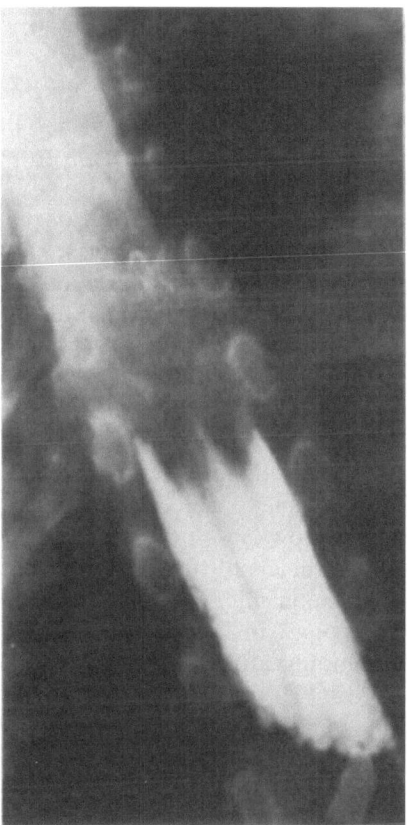

Figure 8.1. Myelography showing complete block with irregular trifid edge at T-11 to T-12. (Reprinted with permission of Adeloye A, Folami AO, Aghadiung PU: Schistosoma haematobium granuloma of the spinal cord in a Nigerian boy. Neurochirurgia 25:100–102, 1982.)

disease and the difficulty of radical excision of the granuloma in the cord or conus medullaris without incurring further neurological damage dictate a combination of conservative surgery and chemotherapy.

In diffuse granulomatosis, a small but carefully selected biopsy should be performed at the time of laminectomy. If the cord is diffusely swollen, the dura should be left open. After laminectomy, bilharzial chemotherapy is given.

The large discrete granuloma requires careful surgery. A radical removal should *not* be carried out when bilharzial disease is suspected, since further and devastating damage to the cord invariably occurs. A large granuloma shrinks with chemotherapy, but the regression takes a long time to occur during which neurological damage may become irreversible. Hence, early laminectomy saves the cord from damage.

Hydatid Disease

Hydatid disease of the spine is a rare entity first described in 1807 by
Chaussier (32,33). The parasitic disease is caused by the larva of *Echinococcus granulosus* and is endemic in southern Europe and other parts of
the world.

Vertebral hydatidosis occurs in less than 1% of patients suffering from
hydatid disease (34–36); nevertheless, it comprises about 50% of the bony
involvement encountered in the parasitic infestation. Spinal hydatid disease
is uncommonly associated with an intracranial lesion (37).

Pathology

Hydatid disease of the bone is always primary and is characterized by a
tendency to infiltrate spongy bone. The occurrence of the larva in the
bone is usually multilocular due to lack of defensive reaction of the tissue.
In the spine the parasite grows in all directions, involving the vertebral
bodies, pedicles, laminae, heads of ribs, and adjacent soft tissue (35,38).

Spinal hydatidosis is responsible for about 2% of all cases of spinal cord
compression in Egypt (39); 4% in Turkey (40); 4.5% in Morocco; and 14%
in Tunisia (41). It commonly affects the thoracic spine (36,42–44); less
often the lumbar, and least so the cervical spine may be affected.

Hydatid cysts of the spine are usually unilateral, raising the possibility
that the parasitic embryo circulating in the bloodstream enters through
an intercostal artery (45).

Clinical Features

More males than females are affected by spinal hydatidosis (35,36,40).
Most of the patients are young, many of them being in the second decade
of life. In a series of 11 patients described in Turkey (40), two were aged
10 and 12 years, respectively.

The slow growth of the disease is responsible for its late presentation.
The main symptoms are related to the occurrence of fracture, infection,
local swelling, and neurological involvement. The first complaint is usually
of radicular pain; the physical signs are those of spinal and radicular
compression. Marked exacerbation of symptoms and signs tends to occur
on palpation or percussion of the spine. About 20% of patients have had
some form of trauma to the spine before the disease (41).

Diagnosis

The clinical diagnosis of spinal hydatidosis is difficult. Even in parts of
the world where the disease is endemic, preoperative diagnosis is made

in less than 50% of cases. Its role as a cause of spinal cord compression should always be borne in mind where hydatid disease is endemic.

Osseous changes, as seen on plain x-ray films of the spine, occur in about 30% of cases (40). In the vertebral bodies, moth-eaten areas surrounded by sclerosis are typical of the disease. Calcifications may extend from the lesion to adjacent soft tissue. Computed tomography (CT) scans of the vertebral bodies often show multiple cystic cavities and bony erosion, all producing a honeycomb appearance. In the majority of cases myelography locates the block (35). The Casoni and Weinberg tests used in the diagnosis of the disease have no useful value if only the bones are affected (40).

Treatment

Surgical treatment is ideal in the presence of spinal cord compression. Laminectomy and extirpation of the cyst is the operation of choice (35,36). In 90% of cases, hydatid cysts are found in the extradural space, usually in association with bony involvement (40). Intradural extramedullary cysts are very rare (41,42,45,46). Other surgical procedures like decompression with anterior vertebrectomy and fusion are less often used.

Spinal hydatidosis is a disease of young adults, hence extensive removal of cancellous bone should be followed by stabilization of the spine with bone grafts (36).

Complete surgical extirpation is not often possible because of extensive tissue invasion by the parasite. About 60% of the patients improve after surgery. Mortality ranges from 3% to 15% and recurrence from 30% to 40% (36,41,42).

Recurrence is rare in intradural extramedullary disease but relatively common in the extradural variety (40). The recurrence tends to occur soon after surgery, leading to repeated operative decompression in most cases. Thus, in the series of Apt et al. (35), the average number of surgical interventions per patient was 2.6. The value of irrigating the surgical field with hypertonic saline to prevent recurrence is not proved (40). The postoperative administration of mebendazole, a drug of proven value in systemic echinococcus disease, may reduce the incidence of recurrence.

Prognosis

This is strongly influenced by the neurological state of the patient at the time of surgery. Hence, surgery should be performed as soon as possible before irreversible cord damage occurs.

The results of treatment are good in the immediate postoperative period, but long-term results are poor (35). Patients often are not cured, but made able to "live with their disease" (34).

Cysticercosis

This is the human infestation caused by the larval form of pork tapeworm *(Taenia solium)*. The ova of the parasite, after ingestion, are carried to various parts of the body where they develop into cysticerci. The common sites of localization are the skin, subcutaneous tissue, skeletal muscles, eyes, heart, and the nervous system. Parasitosis is common in Asia, parts of Europe, Latin America (particularly Mexico), and India.

Although involvement of the brain and its enveloping meninges often occurs, invasion of the spinal cord is comparatively rare (47–50). Thus, of the 450 cases of cysticercosis reported by Dixon and Lipscomb (51), only one showed progressive paraplegia as a result of spinal cord involvement. Also, in 47 cases of cysticercosis of the nervous system examined at autopsy and reported by the same workers (52), the cysticerci were distributed as follows: cerebrum, 44; meninges, 22; cerebellum, 8; and spinal cord, 2.

Pathology

In pathophysiological terms, spinal cysticercosis may be primary or secondary (53). The primary form may present either as an isolated disease or as part of multifocal cysticercosis. The secondary disease may result either from direct spinal extension of a massive intracranial cysticercosis or from cervical pachymeningitis and cord degeneration occurring in posterior fossa cysticercosis.

Three anatomical forms of spinal cysticercosis are recognized: intramedullary, leptomeningeal extramedullary, and extradural extramedullary (51). The rarest form is the extradural variety. The most frequent type is the leptomeningeal disease, which is about six to eight times more common than the intramedullary lesion (54); up to 26 cases of intramedullary cysticercosis have been reported in the literature (54–58). The distribution of intramedullary cysticercosis is related to the blood flow to the cord, suggesting a hematogenous route of infection.

Three mechanisms have been suggested to explain the manifestations of spinal cysticercosis. These are

1. An inflammatory reaction caused by the metabolites of the parasite or the degenerated larval remains (59);
2. Mass effect of intramedullary or extramedullary cyst (54);
3. Cord degeneration caused by pachymeningitis or vascular insufficiency (54,60).

Diagnosis

Males are more affected than females. All age-groups are susceptible to spinal cysticercosis, but it is more common in adults than in children.

The patient often presents with back pain and difficulty in walking and in passing urine. Paraplegia is usually progressive and associated with a sensory level. Myelography usually shows a block. The disease should be considered in the differential diagnosis of cord compression in areas of the world where cysticercosis is common.

Treatment

Laminectomy is the treatment of choice and its results are satisfactory (49).

Dracunculiasis (Guinea Worm Infestation) of the Spine

Infestation by *Dracunculus medinensis,* a common parasitic disease in Africa and Asia, may involve the nervous system. Except for the four cases reported in India—one by Donaldson and Angelo (61), one by Mathur et al. (62), and two by Reddy and Valli (63)—the documentation of guinea worm infestation of the spine has come largely from Africa. This includes six cases from Nigeria (64,65), three from the Ivory Coast (66), two from Ghana (67), and one from Niger (68). There have also been a few isolated case reports (69,70).

Pathology

Although it is known that the guinea worm can migrate freely in the retroperitoneal space, it is not certain how it reaches the spinal cord. Settling in the extradural space, the parasite provokes a low-grade inflammatory process and segmental cord ischemia, resulting in limb paralysis. The site most commonly involved is T-4 to T-8, this being the level of critical vascular anastomosis where any ischemic process can severely and acutely damage the cord. The cervical spine is rarely involved.

Clinical Features

Limb weakness is usually of sudden onset. Sphincter disturbance follows the paralysis. In some cases fever may be present. A sensory level is commonly demonstrated on physical examination.

The diagnosis is rarely made clinically, since guinea worm paraplegia does not characteristically differ from other causes of paraplegia seen where guinea worm is endemic. The differential diagnosis of guinea worm paraplegia include Burkitt's lymphoma, pyogenic spine abscess, tuberculosis of the spine, and other parasitic infestations of the spine.

Most of the cases of guinea worm abscess were diagnosed after exploration of the spine. The disease should be suspected in paraplegia of sudden onset encountered in a patient from an area where guinea worm is endemic.

A history of infection with discharge of worms from unusual extraspinal and multiple sites reinforces the suspicion.

Investigation

Peripheral eosinophilia or eosinophilic hyperplasia of the bone marrow occurs in some patients.

Plain radiograph findings of the spine are usually normal; in some cases paravertebral calcification in a dead worm is seen (62). A frontal CT scan of the normal spine is sometimes useful. It may reveal calcification within the spinal canal (68). The most useful diagnostic procedure is myelography. It may show either partial extradural block with deviation of the column in early cases or a complete block in late cases. Iophendylate has been used as the contrast material in most cases, but metrizamide is better.

A combination of tomography and myelography enabled Legmann et al. (68) to diagnose the disease in their patient.

Treatment

Laminectomy is the treatment of choice, with about 50% of the patients recovering after the operation. The worm is often recovered from the extradural compartment (71). When laminectomy is performed late, cord recovery is poor. Apart from the duration of the disease, other factors affect the prognosis, as some cases subjected to early laminectomy did not recover from the effects of cord compression in the series of Khwaja et al. (64). A course of niridazole, which is specific for guinea worm, and broad-spectrum antibiotics to control any super-added infection should be administered. Odaibo et al. (65) favour the use of metronidazole and tetracycline in early cases of spinal dracontiasis.

Paragonimiasis

Human paragonimiasis has been reported in South America and in parts of Africa. An outbreak of the disease occurred in Eastern Nigeria during the Nigeria Civil War (72). The parasitic infestation is due to the lung fluke, *Paragonimus*. Improperly cooked crabs or cray fish infested with the larval stage (metacercariae) of the parasite are responsible for the disease. *Paragonimus westermani* causes the disease in South America; the species responsible for the disease in Africa is not known for sure.

Clinical Features and Treatment

It is a disease of young people, with about 75% of the patients being under the age of 20 years. Respiratory symptoms are the common presentation.

Extrapulmonary disease, particularly involvement of the central nervous system, is rare. Invasion of the spinal cord is thought to occur directly and is therefore less amenable to surgical treatment. Bithionol, the drug of choice, is useful in cases of spinal cord paragonimiasis.

References

1. Bilharz T: Further observations concerning Distomum haematobium in the portal vein of man and its relationship to certain pathological formation. Z Wiss Zool 4:72–76, 1853.
2. Dar J, Zimmerman RR: Schistosomiasis of the spinal cord. Surg Neurol 8: 416–418, 1977.
3. Luyendijk W, Lindeman J: Schistosomiasis (Bilharziasis) mansoni of the spinal cord simulating an intramedullary tumour. Surg Neurol 4:457–60, 1975.
4. Norfray JF, Schlachter L, Heiser WJ, et al: Schistosomiasis of the spinal cord. Surg Neurol 9:68–71, 1978.
5. Levy LF, Baldachin BJ, Clain D: Intracranial bilharzia. Cent Afr J Med 21: 76–84, 1975.
6. Herskowitz A: Spinal cord involvement with schistosoma mansoni. J Neurosurg 36:494–498, 1972.
7. Odeku EL, Lucas AO, Richard DR: Intramedullary spinal cord schistosomiasis. J Neurosurg 29:417–423, 1968.
8. Adeloye A, Folami AO, Aghadiung PU: Schistosoma haematobium granuloma of the spinal cord in a Nigerian boy. Neurochirurgia 25:100–102, 1982.
9. Ruberti RF, Chopra SA: Schistosomiasis of the spinal cord. Med Afr Noire 23:77–81, 1976.
10. Batson OV: The function of the vertebral veins and their role in the spread of metastases. Ann Surg 112:138–149, 1940.
11. Kane CA, Most H: Schistosomiasis of the central nervous system: experiences in World War 2 and review of the literature. Arch Neurol Psychiat 59:141–183, 1948.
12. Marciel Z, Coelho B, Abath G: Myelite schistosomique due au S. mansoni. Rev Neurol 91:241–259, 1954.
13. Cohen J, Capildeo R, Clifford-Rose F, et al: Schistosomal myelopathy. Br Med J 1:1258, 1977.
14. Budzilovich GN, Most H, Feigin I: Pathogenesis and latency of spinal cord schistosomiasis. Arch Pathol 77:383–388, 1964.
15. Abbott PH, Spencer H: Transverse myelitis due to ova of schistosoma mansoni. Trans Soc Trop Med Hyg 47:221–223, 1953.
16. Gelfand M: A clinical study of intestinal bilharziasis in Africa. London: Edward Arnold, 1967.
17. Hutton PW, Holland HT: Schistosomiasis of the spinal cord. Br Med J 2: 1931–33, 1960.
18. Faust EC: An inquiry into the ectopic lesions in schistosomiasis. Am J Trop Med 28:175, 1948.
19. Marcial-Rojas RA, Fiol RE: Neurological complications of schistosomiasis. Ann Intern Med 59:215–230, 1963.
20. Wakefield GS, Carroll JD, Speed DE: Schistosomiasis of the spinal cord. Brain 85:535–52, 1962.

21. Gelfand M: Schistosomiasis in South Central Africa. Juta, Cape Town, 1950.
22. Levy LF: Bilharzial involvement of the central nervous system. Med J Zambia 4:191, 1970.
23. El Banhawy A, Zidan A, El-Kader G: Bilharziasis of the spinal cord. J Egypt Surg Soc 5:160, 1970.
24. Barnett AM: Bilharzial granuloma of the spinal cord. S Afr Med J 39:699–700, 1965.
25. Bird AV: Spinal cord complications of bilharziasis. S Afr Med J 39:158–162, 1965.
26. El-Banhawy A: Bilharziasis of the spinal cord. Rev Neurol Neurocir Psiquiatr 40:43, 1978.
27. Rée GH: Central neurological syndromes caused by parasites. Medicine Digest 12 (2):4–8, 1986.
28. Levy LF, Taube E: Two further cases of spinal bilharziasis. Cent Afr J Med 15:52, 1969.
29. Dunston THJ, Pepler WJ: A new complement fixation test for schistosomiasis. S Afr Med J 39:162, 1965.
30. Ghaly AE: El Banhawy A: Schistosomiasis of the spinal cord. J Pathol 111:57–60, 1973.
31. Molyneux ME, Galatius-Jensen F: Successful drug treatment of schistosomal myelopathy. A case report. S Afr Med J 54:871–872, 1978.
32. Chaussier: Compression of upper thoracic spinal cord by Echinococcus cyst. J Med Chir Pharmacol 14:231–37, 1807.
33. Rayport M, Wisoff HS, Zaiman H: Vertebral echinococcus. J Neurosurg 21:647–59, 1964.
34. Fitzpatrick SC: Hydatid disease of the lumbar vertebrae. J Bone Joint Surg 47B:286–291, 1965.
35. Apt WL, Fierro JL, Calderon C, et al: Vertebral hydatid disease. Clinical experience with 27 cases. J Neurosurg 44:72–76, 1976.
36. Turtas S, Viale ES, Pau A: Long-term results of surgery for hydatid disease of the spine. Surg Neurol 13:468–470, 1980.
37. Carrea R, Dowling E, Guevara JA: Surgical treatment of hydatid cysts of the central nervous system in the paediatric age. Childs Brain 1:4–22, 1975.
38. Arana-Iniguez R, Lopez-Fernandez JR: Parasitosis of the nervous system with special reference to echinococcus. Clin Neurosurg 4:123–144, 1967.
39. Sorour O, Rifaat M, Lofti M, et al: Spinal cord compression—ten years experience. Med J Cairo 45:339–345, 1977.
40. Pamir MN, Akalan N, Ozgen T, et al: Spinal hydatid cysts. Surg Neurol 21:53–7, 1984.
41. Bettaieb A, Khaldi T, Ben Rhonma T, et al: L'echinococcose vertébro-médullaire. Neurochirurgie 24:205–10, 1978.
42. Acquaviva R, Tamic PM: L'echinococcose vertébromédullaire. A propos de 14 observations. Neurochirurgie 10:649–50, 1964.
43. Morshed AA: Hydatid disease of spine. Neurochirurgia 20:211–15, 1977.
44. Robinson RG: Hydatid disease of the spine and its neurological complication. Br J Surg 47:301–6, 1959.
45. Ley A, Marti A: Intramedullary hydatic cyst. J Neurosurg 33:257–9, 1970.

46. Sharma A, Kashyap V, Abraham J, et al: Intradural hydatid cysts. Surg Neurol 16:235–7, 1981.
47. Dixon HBF, Smithers DW: Epilepsy in cysticercosis. Q J Med 3:603–616, 1934.
48. MacArthur WP: Cysticercosis as seen in the British Army with special reference to the production of epilepsy. Trans R Soc Trop Med Hyg 27:343–363, 1934.
49. Natarajan M, Ramasubramanian KR, Muthu AK: Intramedullary cysticercosis of spinal cord. Surg Neurol 6:157–8, 1976.
50. Stern WE: Neurosurgical considerations of cysticercosis of the central nervous system. J Neurosurg 55:382–389, 1981.
51. Dixon HBF, Lipscomb FM: Cysticercosis: an analysis and follow up of 450 cases. Spec Rep Sev Med Res Counc Lond 299:1–58, 1961.
52. Roy RN, Bhattacharya MB, Chatterjee BP, et al: Spinal cysticercosis. Surg Neurol 6:129–131, 1976.
53. Akiguchi I, Fujiwara T, Matsuyama H, et al: Intramedullary spinal cysticercosis. Neurology 29:1531–34, 1979.
54. Queiroz LDS, Filho AP, Callegaro D: Intramedullary cysticercosis. J Neurol Sci 26:61–70, 1975.
55. Cabieses F, Vallenas M, Landa R: Cysticercosis of the spinal cord. J Neurosurg 16:337–341, 1959.
56. Mehta DS, Malik GB, Dar J: Intramedullary cysticercosis. Neurol India 19: 92–94, 1971.
57. Singh A, Aggarwal ND, Malhotra KC, et al: Spinal cysticercosis with paraplegia. Br Med J 2:684–5, 1966.
58. Garza-Mercado R: Intramedullary cysticercosis. Surg Neurol 5:331–332, 1976.
59. Greenfield JG, Blackwood W, McMenemey WH: Neuropathology. London: Edward Arnold, 1958, pp 215–217.
60. Kahn P: Cysticercosis of the central nervous system with amyotrophic lateral sclerosis. J Neurol Neurosurg Psychiatr 35:81–87, 1972.
61. Donaldson JR, Angelo TA: Quadriplegia due to guinea worm abscess. J Bone Joint Surg [AM] 43:197, 1961.
62. Mathur PPS, Dharker SR, Hiran S, et al: Lumbar extradural compression by guinea worm infestation. Surg Neurol 17:127–9, 1982.
63. Reddy CRRM, Valli VV: Extradural guinea worm abscess. Report of two cases. Am J Trop Med Hyg 16:23, 1967.
64. Khwaja NS, Dosseter JFB, Lawrie JH: Extradural guinea worm abscess. J Neurosurg 43:627, 1975.
65. Odaibo SK, Awogun IA, Oshagbemi K: Paraplegia complicating dracontiasis. J R Coll Surg Edin 31:376–378, 1986.
66. Giordano C, Kanga K, Doucet J, et al: Compression médullaire par filaire de médine: à propos de 3 cas. Med Afr Noire 23:83, 1976.
67. Mitra AK, Haddock DRW: Paraplegia due to guinea worm infestation. Trans R Soc Trop Med Hyg 64:102, 1970.
68. Legmann P, Chiras J, Launay M, et al: Epidural dracunculiasis: a rare cause of spinal cord compression. Neuroradiology 20:43, 1980.
69. Chakroun M: Localisation exceptionelle de la filaire de médine (à propos d'une observation d'abcès de l'espace épidural). Thèse Méd Paris, 1963.

70. Margairaz A, Rosier M, Schneider J, et al: Complication neurologique inédite de la filariose. Rev Neurol (Paris) 108:59, 1963.
71. Adeloye A: Extradural compression by guinea worm. Surg Neurol 19:482, 1983.
72. Nwokolo C: Outbreak of paragonimiasis in Eastern Nigeria. Lancet 1: 32–33, 1972.

CHAPTER 9

Diagnostics and Management of Urinary Problems in Neurogenic Vesico-Sphincteric Dysfunction

Gérard Monfort

Neurogenic vesicosphincteric dysfunction of the lower urinary tract occurs not only in patients with congenital malformations of neurologic origin, but also in patients with less significant neurologic disturbances such as diabetes, anemia and sclerosis.

However congenital malformations of the spine are the most important cause of such a dysfunction in childhood, and a significant proportion of upper and lower urinary tract diseases is secondary to vesical and sphincteric dysfunction. Pyelonephritis, urinary tract infection (UTI) and urinary incontinence are the most likely to occur in such pathologic conditions. A knowledge of the mechanism of normal micturition and recognition of these abnormalities are essential for the diagnosis and treatment of these forms of uropathology.

Were herein present:

1. A brief approach to the function of the lower urinary tract and its relation to neuropathology.
2. Description of specific diagnostic procedures.
3. Urinary function evolution in the meningomyelocele patient.
4. Treatment of vesico-neurogenic dysfunction in infancy.

Normal Pathologic Concepts

The human bladder is composed of three main structures, which are totally different in embryologic origin, vascularisation, innervation and function are concerned. Although different, it is the complete synergy and complex interconnection of the three that make normal functioning of the lower urinary tract possible, thus permitting:

1. storage of urine
2. passive continence
3. and the normal micturition mechanism.

It is an abnormality of the neurologic control of the normal anatomic structures that are responsible for the so-called "neurologic bladder" which is, in fact, a vesico-sphincteric dysfunction of neurologic origin.

These structures are known as the detrusor, trigone, and external sphincter. The lower urinary tract stores urine at low pressure and periodically expels it. The bladder behaves both as a reservoir and as a pump, while the urethra is closed during filling but opens and becomes a compliant conduit during voiding. This is possible by association of three interrelated and adjacent structures, whose synergic function permits evacuation and continence in normal conditions.

Detrusor (D): endodermic origin para-sympathetic innervation, compliance and storage function, contracts during micturition.

Trigone (T): internal sphincterendo and mesodermic origin, sympathetic innervation. Responsible for passive continence—opens actively during micturition.

External sphincter (S): mesodermic origin, somatic innervation, voluntary and reflex functions. Responsible for active continence.

Detrusor: Storage

The normal vesical response to filling is a slow upward deflection in pressure seen on continuous monitoring (cystometrography). This is mainly a basic property of the vesical wall and does not change immediately after sacral root ablation or decerebration (5).

However, with time, the tone becomes greater than normal and the bladder becomes trabeculated (Fig. 9.1), suggesting that a reflex neural process may serve to moderate the vesical tone when filling and facilitate bladder storage in a normal state. Trabeculation either after decentralization or of a congenital origin probably indicates a compensating hypertrophy of the detrusor muscle and is generally associated with an increase in bladder outlet resistance in the face of dyssynergic expulsive activity. It must be understood as being a local process probably secondary to permanent stimulation of myofibrillary activity induced by an intravesical pressure process.

In addition, selected drugs that cause filling after sacral denervation, such as bethanechol chloride used in the Lapides denervation supra-sensitivity test (DSST) influence the detrusor and increase the tonic response as if there were a hypersensitivity to acetylcholine. On the contrary, anticholinergic agents decrease the tone, indicating an effect on the intrinsic bladder myotonal unit.

In addition to the influence of cholinergic agents on the vesical tone after decentralization, sympathetics and antagonists affect the detrusor response to filling. Both alpha- and beta-receptors are present in detrusor and urethral smooth musculature. It has been demonstrated that alpha-receptors are relatively abundant in the trigone, and that beta-receptors

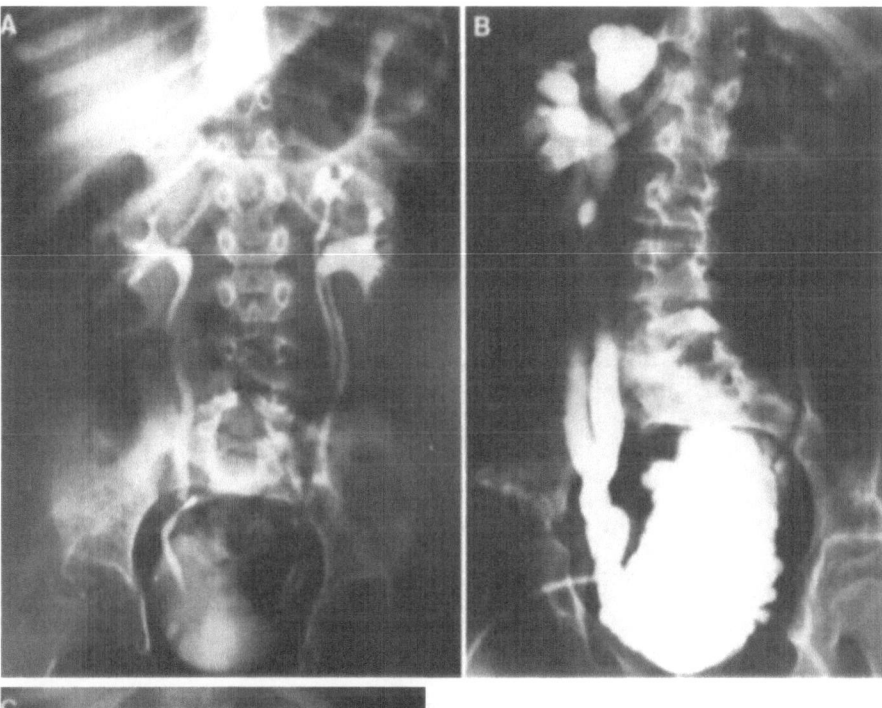

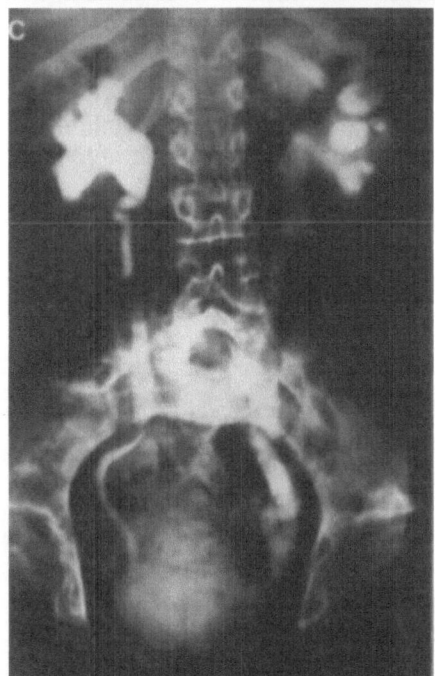

Figure 9.1. Spontaneous evolution of the bladder toward trabeculation: **A** age 7; **B, C** age 15. Note the difference between the hypertonic and spastic detrusor (D +) and the flaccid, paralyzed trigone (T −) in **B**.

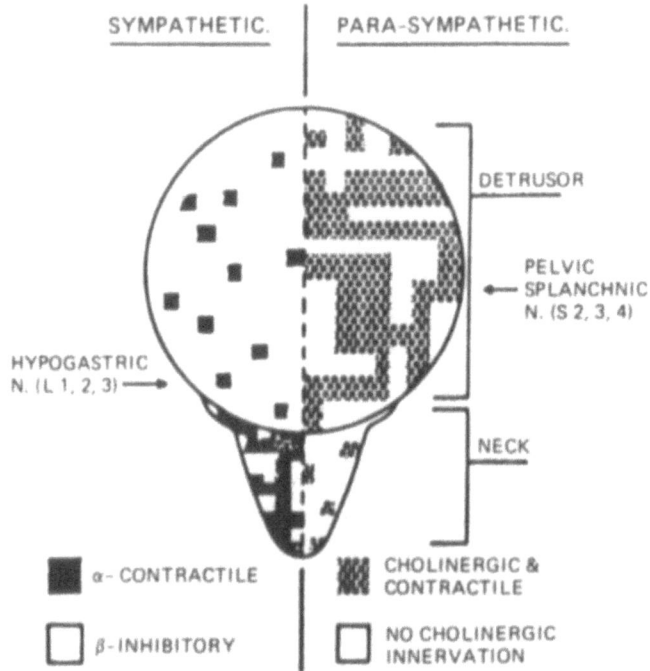

Figure 9.2. Alpha- and beta-receptor distribution in a normal bladder.

are found in the bladder body (Fig. 9.2). If sympathetic stimulation is applied during bladder filling, the urethral smooth muscle contracts but the bladder muscle relaxes. However, it has been established that this activity is modified by efferent and probably afferent pelvic nerves and sacral cord activity.

Trigone: Passive Continence

Continence is normally maintained by the preservation of urethral pressure which is higher than that of the bladder. Urine is normally held at the vesical outlet. This depends on the smooth-muscle internal urethral sphincter (trigonal-cervical complex or bladder neck), and is not affected by a bilateral pudendal nerve loss.

It is clear that a malformation of the cauda equina such as that encountered in meningomyelocele or sacral agenesis, is associated with incontinence. In fact the detrusor pressure becomes abnormal and, despite maintenance of urethral closing pressure, incontinence occurs as a result of an intrinsic vesical response to filling. This ultimately pushes urine across the internal sphincter (closed only by smooth-muscular activity). If this function is lost, incontinence is quite severe despite the preservation of considerable urethral closing pressure exerted on the urethra by the activity of the skeletal musculature.

Moreover, the internal sphincter, because of its intra-abdominal position is given a mechanical advantage over the external sphincter, which must actively compress the urethra as changes in intra-abdominal pressure are transmitted directly to the internal sphincter, and indirectly to the external sphincter.

The closure of the urethra by smooth muscular counteractivity is partly the result of constant sympathetic tonus. However, there is a definite influence exerted by pelvic nerve activity, both afferent and efferent, on urethral receptor response. This is demonstrated by the effect of alpha-adrenergic blocking agents which may create a loss of function or a smooth muscular hypofunction as is sometimes encountered in pathologic conditions.

External Sphincter: Active Continence

The external sphincter is subject to volitional control, but also has some unique characteristics of its own. The tone persists in all circumstances except micturition and defecation, and recruitment occurs reflexively with standing, coughing, and during vesical filling. Contraction of the sphincter is associated with direct inhibition of the detrusor motor neuron within the spinal cord.

Cortical impulse conveyed by the pyramidal tract can induce a contraction of the external sphincter and stop micturition, even after it has begun. This effect is voluntary. Conversely, the first effect in volitionally directed micturition is relaxation of the pelvic floor and external sphincter, and this is a totally reflex mechanism. However, the fact that the external and internal sphincters normally work together tends to prove that the pudendal nerve has an influence on intrinsic skeletal sphincter activity. Electromyography recorded from the anal sphincter usually reflects the urethral striated sphincter activity (at least in normal conditions), but this can be doubtful in some pathologic conditions.

Spinal Innervation and Micturition Center

The detrusor motor cells have been found in the intermediolateralis columns of conus medullaris, from S2 to S4. The pudendal motor neurons responsible for the innervation of sacral roots and pelvic floor are located in Onuf's nucleus (anterior horn of the sacral cord segments).

The intermediolateralis columns from T-10 to L-2 contain the neurons concerned with sympathetic innervation of the bladder, sphincter, and male genitals. Finally, there does not seem to be a true micturition center. Transection of the spine results in loss of the normal sequence. Afferent activity generated by bladder filling projects directly to the brainstem of

the cat, suggesting that the "center" is supraspinal. Inhibitory and facil-
itatory centers have been described experimentally.

DTS Synergia: Normal Micturition Mechanism

At certain bladder pressures filling and reflex detrusor contraction are
elicited. This event involves peripheral, spinal and supraspinal neural activity, but the end result is a coordinated increase in intravesical pressure
with a decrease in intraurethral pressure and relaxation of pelvic floor
musculation. This complex of activity continues until complete vesical
emptying occurs and depends on the normal brainstem.

This micturition can be looked upon as a triple circuit affair: distension
of the bladder results in impulses being sent along different pathways via
the pelvic nerves to the sacral spinal cord. Internuncial neurons in the
cord allow stimulation of parasympathetic, sympathetic (at the thoracolumbar level) and somatic efferent fibers that travel to the DTS system.

Frontal and parietal lobe communications may act to facilitate or inhibit
these efferent spinal cord pathways. It is conjectured that these pathways
are present and intact (although not completely myelinated) in the newborn
and coordinated activity between D and T + S is present when bladder
emptying takes place. During the first two years of life, however, bladder
capacity enlarges slowly as the brainstem inhibitory center acts to control
micturition. Maturation of the frontal and parietal lobes also progresses,
first with the awareness of bladder fullness, then with the ability to inhibit
voiding, and finally to facilitate it.

DTS Dyssynergia (Fig. 9.2)

Each component of the DTS association can respond independently from
the two others and, therefore, many combinations are theoretically possible. Detrusor alteration is responsible for hypertonicity, giving hypertension and stasis in the upper tract. On the contrary, detrusor paralysis
gives a low pressure reservoir and protects it. Trigone and internal
sphincter can be paralysed. One of the consequences might be the destruction of normal antireflux mechanism. Incontinence will be complete.
But they are more rarely spastic and closed, thus giving retention and
overflow incontinence.

The external sphincter is the most affected of the three elements. When
unpaired its evolution is similar to other paraplegic muscles, that is toward
spasticity and fibrosis, thus causing bladder outlet resistance. The spastic
external sphincter creates a typical obstructive uropathy, the evolution
of which in the past resulted in renal insufficiency and death in young
adulthood. Early treatment was directed toward either destruction
(sphincterotomies) or bypass (permanent urinary diversion).

Diagnostic Procedures

There is a major difference in the diagnostic procedures between the adult and child population. In the adult group, most of the patients had at one time normal micturition, and they are able to describe inadequacy of micturition sequence, as well as incontinence. Conversely, most children affected with congenital neurogenic dysfunction have never had normal, physiologic, complete emptying of the lower urinary tract and, as far as continence is concerned, have few points of reference with normality. Moreover, there is a wide spectrum of urologic conditions induced by neurologic dysfunction which are not stable over time and add their pathology to the already destroyed system, such as massive reflux or urinary tract infection.

Clinical Evaluation

It is impossible to determine precisely the onset and evolution of urinary tract deterioration by clinical evaluation alone. It is generally admitted that the worse the neurologic condition, the worse the urologic condition. Note must be made of the history of birth and development, the patterns of incontinence, bowel and bladder habits. Spine and lower extremities must be carefully examined for reflex loss, muscle mass, gait, and perineal sensation, tone and reflex (bulbocavernous). However, it must be clear that a neurologic examination of the very young child is difficult because it requires accurate evaluation of subjective responses that the baby is not able to give even in normal conditions, because of the nondevelopment of myelinated fibers in the spine at this age. This must be routinely complemented by a radiographic evaluation of the spine, with special attention given to the sacrum. Loss of sacral roots can be correlated with sacral anomalies. They are highly suggestive of neurologic dysfunction of the lower urinary tract.

Intravenous Pyelography and Sonographic Examination

Intravenous pyelography has long been the most useful and simple examination. It provides indirect information of renal blood flow and renal, pyelocaliceal and ureteral physiopathology. Any deterioration of the lower tract will immediately affect the upper tract. However, intravenous pyelography can actually be replaced by renal ultrasound which is less invasive, well tolerated by patients and family, and completed by a DTPA scan when deterioration occurs. This has the advantage of demonstrating separate right and left kidney function if some therapeutic approach is needed.

Voiding Cystouretrography

This examination is used not only to detect vesicoureteral reflux, but also to analyze detrusor contractions, bladder outlet aspect and to give an approximation regarding the level of an obstructive process. It must be done as soon as possible, before any surgical approach to the neurologic malformation (Fig. 9.3) and is an essential part of the evaluation of infants when there is an indication for treatment. A suprapubic approach is less dangerous than retrograde filling, and careful attention must be given to any symptoms that are present at birth in 6% to 10% of the cases. For instance, detrusor external sphincter dyssynergia is easily recognized since the proximal urethra and bladder neck are widely dilated while the mid- or membranous urethra is tightly compressed (Fig. 9.4).

A simple upright cystogram provides information about the continence mechanism. Normally the bladder neck is closed. If this area is open from the start of filling, then a deficit in urethral smooth muscular continence function exists. The association of cystography and simple cystometry (either with a number 6 or number 8 catheter, or a double catheter) can be done without the use of a sophisticated monitoring system, and adds

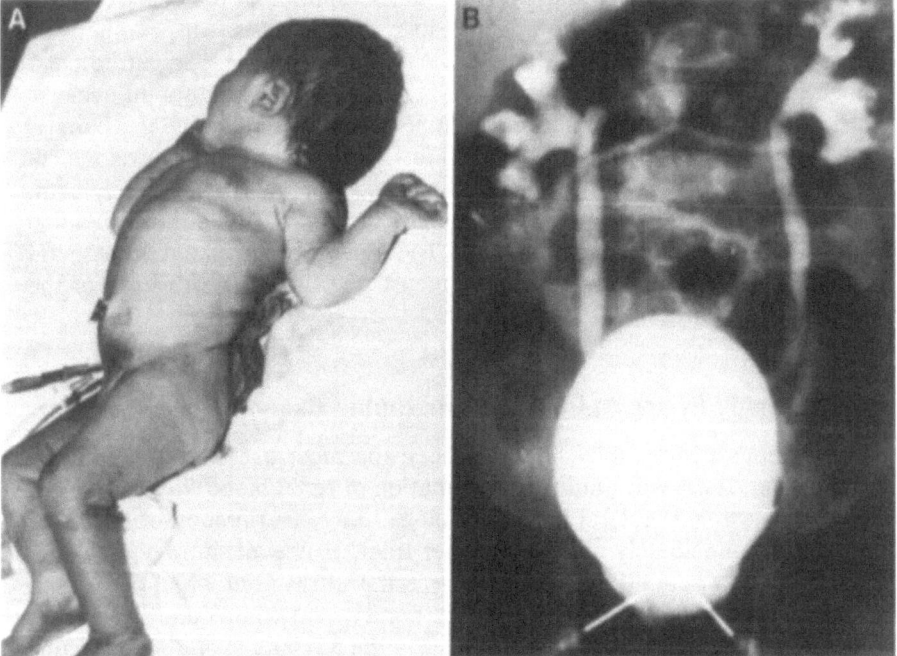

Figure 9.3. A Suprapubic cystogram at birth. Note the presence of the lesion on the back. **B** Result: smooth bladder. Bilasteral stage 3 vesicoureteral reflux.

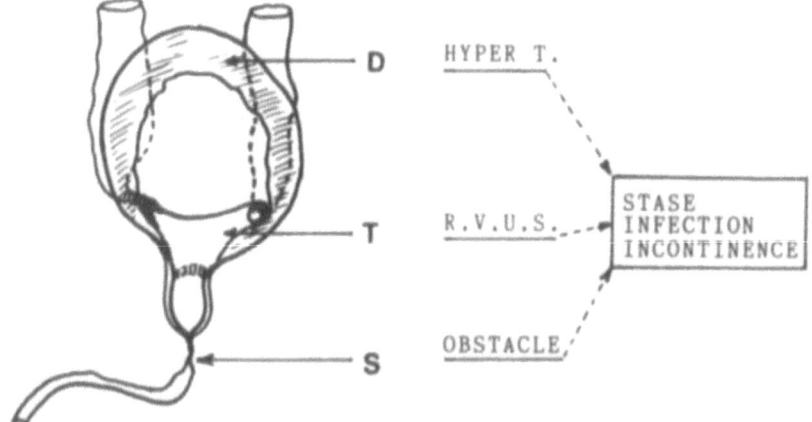

Figure 9.4. DTS system and its relationship to pathology. R.V.U.S.: secondary vesicoureteral reflux.

to a static examination of all the information given by the urodynamic assessment (Figs. 9.5, 9.6). The 10 × 10 camera spot film gives a dynamic approach to most of the urologic consequences of a neurogenic dysfunction such as diverticula, vesicoureteral reflux, trabeculated bladder, detrusor hyperactivity or atony, internal sphincter decompensation and the like.

Urodynamics

The diagnosis of uncoordinated bladder sphincter contraction can be difficult to make without the help of EMG of the pelvic floor. In fact, urodynamic studies in children consist of a normal voiding cystouretrography as well as an EMG. This can be elaborated by adding an intraabdominal (rectal) pressure study and an intraurethral study, but one may doubt the real value of this assessment in a not perfectly cooperative patient, which is usually the case for children (Fig. 9.7). Urinary flow rate studies, urethral profile pressure studies, and endoscopic diagnostics have been of no use in this particular age group, at least in our experience.

Classification of Neuropathic Bladder

Attempts to adapt the adult neurologic classification to children has failed to demonstrate any real value for three major reasons: a) congenital lesion means no previous normality, b) maturation of an abnormal system is not encountered in an adult, and c) pathologic evolution proceeds for decades.

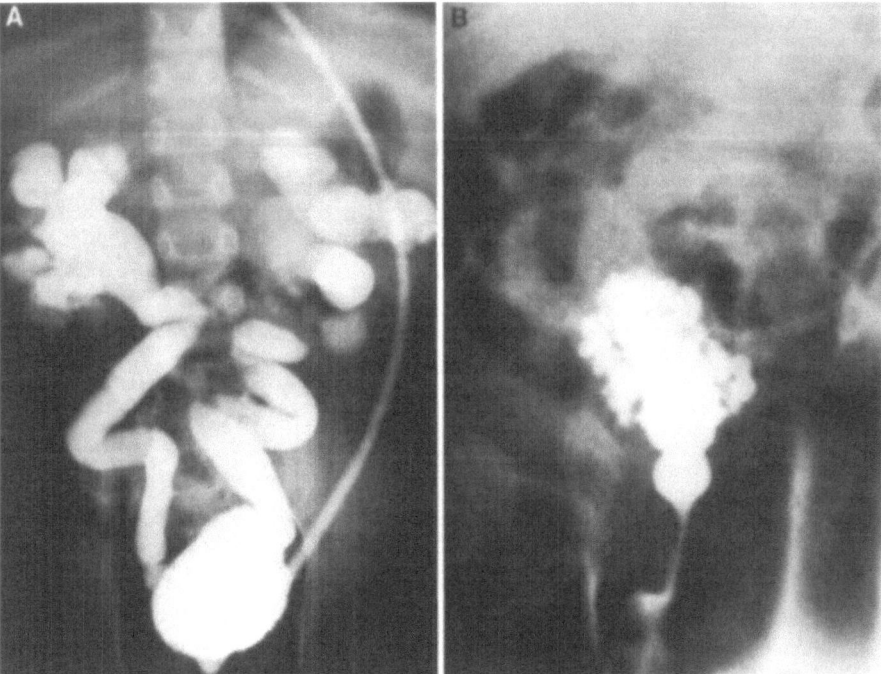

Figure 9.5. A Massive reflux in a baby. Note also the paralyzed trigone; bladder neck open. **B** Severe deterioration (present at birth) in a baby girl. The detrusor is trabeculated and full of saccules and diverticulas. The bladder neck is widely opened, and the posterior urethra is dilated on a spastic external sphincter.

A more convenient urologic approach has been proposed and adopted by most pediatric urologists, and is based on the dysfunction of a specific area of the vesicoureteral unit rather than on a specific etiology and related to DTS system. This is known as "storage evacuation" system.

Improper storage may be related to the alteration of detrusor function (D) or inadequate urethral closure mechanism (T). The bladder may have increased tone either by overactivity from excessive or unopposed sympathetic discharge or hyperflexia due to a central nervous system lesion above the sacral cord that prevents the normal inhibitory centers from influencing the sacral reflex arc. Alternatively, incontinence may occur with any one of these conditions, when the bladder neck and external sphincter areas do not provide adequate resistance during filling. Incomplete filling of the bladder may be due to hypoactive or areflexive detrusor muscle (D−). However, nonsynchronous relaxation of the bladder neck of the external sphincter (T + S +) (trigone +, sphincter +) can produce a similar effect.

Myogenic failure occurs at the detrusor muscle level which becomes hypertrophic and decompensates owing to persistant outflow resistance.

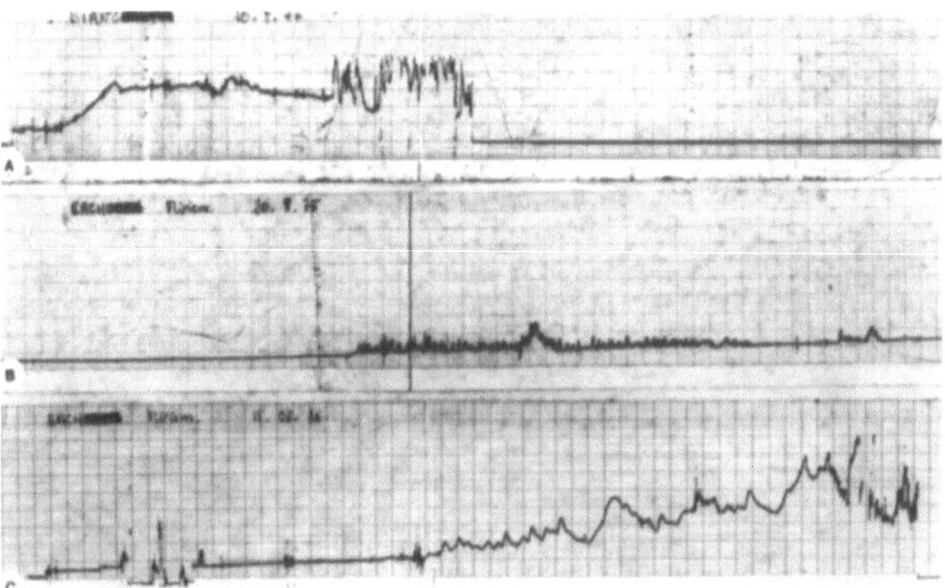

Figure 9.6. Cystometry. **A** Hypertonic bladder with a very high pressure for small volume. **B** Hypotonic bladder (low pressure for high volume). **C** Evolution of **B** toward hypertonicity in 6 months.

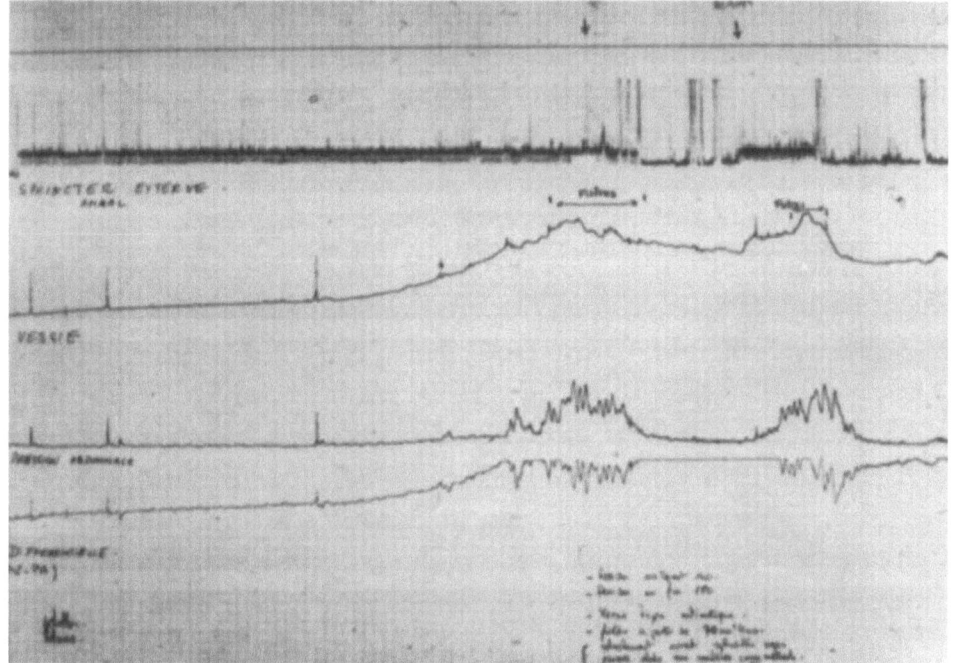

Figure 9.7. Urodynamic study of a neurogenic bladder.

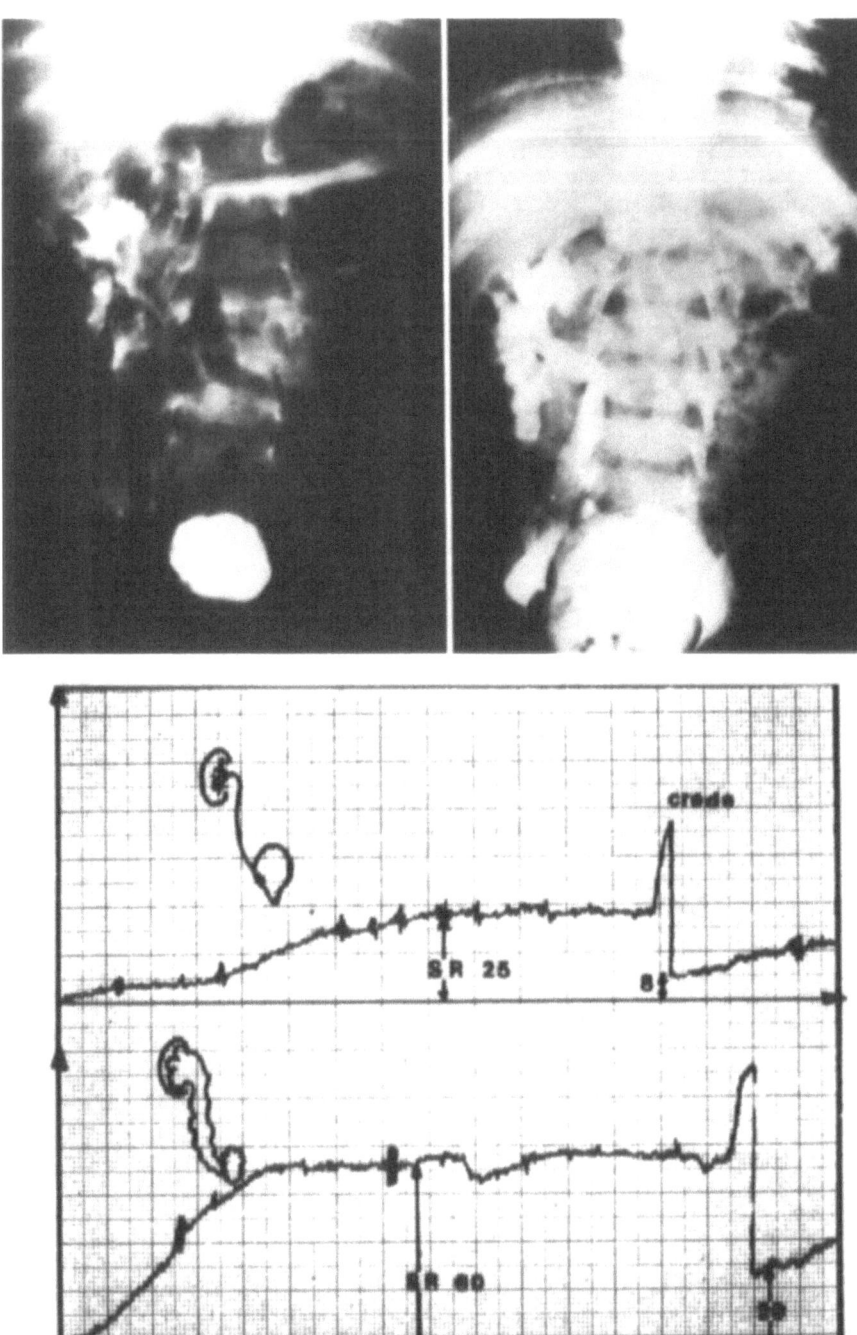

Figure 9.8. Six-month evolution of upper urinary tract in a baby whose first examination showed SR = 40 cm of water (solitary kidney). Relationship of sphincter resistance evolution to urinary tract deterioration.

The major factor seems to be spastic evolution of the external sphincter mechanism, the speed of which is unpredictable.

It is of importance to get an early evaluation of sphincter resistance (SR) for it seems to be the major factor regarding progressive urinary tract deterioration. This SR can easily be measured by reading the pressure in the bladder when the patient begins to leak during a cystometrographic examination; it is a reliable method of predicting the severity and speed of evolution. If the SR is high, destruction of the bladder and distension of the upper tract are likely to occur within a few months (Fig. 9.8).

In childhood, these conditions are encountered in meningomyelocele, lipomeningocele and other occult dysraphysms: tethered cord syndrome, sacral agenesis, cerebral palsy, detrusor hyperreflexia and idiopathic neurogenic bladder.

Evolution of Urinary Tract in Myelodysplasia

A perfect example of evolution of a urinary tract dysfunction in congenital neurologic bladder is illustrated by MMC patients. More than 300 such patients have been followed over a period of 20 years in our institution. They will be used as material for the following considerations. The incidence is 1 per 1000 live births in continental Europe.

Meningomyelocele is not a urinary tract malformation. The urinary tract deterioration is a secondary process occuring in a previously normal urinary tract. Anatomical anomalies are exceptional in that particular group of patients or at least at the same level as that of the normal population. All these patients have had at one point a normal bladder and upper tract. Secondary deterioration is due to dysfunction of the synergic DTS system, and the speed of evolution is closely related to the presence of a neurologic abnormality rather than an anatomic malformation. However, with time, anatomic deterioration such as secondary vesicoureteral reflux, bladder diverticula, or detrusor hypertrophy may appear as specific urologic problems and one may be concerned about their treatment, no matter what the etiology may be.

Only 6% to 10% of newborn babies with MMC are born with an existing deterioration of the urinary tract; 90% have a perfectly normal bladder and upper tract, although abnormally functional. However, the same population 5 years later will proceed, if untreated in the reverse situation, 90% presenting with stasis, distension, infection, incontinence and only 10% still presenting no deterioration, 2% of these will be having normal function.

It is absolutely essential to try to determine, as soon as possible, which children are at risk for deterioration. It has been our impression that it is possible, with the use of early cystometrography (CMG) to single out two factors as being responsible for early deterioration: a) detrusor hypertonicity and hyperactivity (related to high sphincteric resistance), and b) detrusor sphincter dyssynergia (present to a greater or lesser degree in the vast majority of patients). Both conditions may be associated with various degrees of secondary vesicoureteral reflux leading to UTI, usually symptomatic (accute pyelonephritis), and to kidney damage. To diagnose and prevent such conditions diagnostic procedures must be initiated at birth (prior to MMC closure if possible) and then repeated periodically, depending upon the result of the first examination. If the first examination is normal prior to closure, it is exceptional to find abnormalities immediately afterward. Spinal shock seems to be an exceptional phenomenon. However, it is usually difficult to determine if the baby has normal micturition. In this case, taking into consideration the other problems the family is going to be faced with (such as a ventriculoperitoneal shunt, foot and hip mobilization), we usually postpone the problem for a 6-month period, when the examination will be repeated and conditions for emptying and bladder capacity will be explained to the family, together with simple physiotherapy concepts.

If the first examination is abnormal it may be so under two circumstances: a) there are no radiologic changes but CMG shows hypertonicity or hyperactivity and b) both radiographic and CMG abnormalities are present with or without reflux.

In these cases, appropriate treatment must be initiated at once and controls of both anatomic and physiologic conditions repeated each year. However, as soon as the problems encountered have been evaluated and treated as urologic conditions, and the purely neurologic aspect has been reduced to a simple baseline, great progress will have been achieved in the management of this difficult group of patients.

Treatment

The primary goals of the treatment are to ensure periodic emptying of the bladder and to treat hypertonicity and hyperactivity, UTI, low and high-grade vesicoureteral reflux, upper-tract deterioration and incontinence. The different methods of treatment available are medical, physiotherapy and surgery.

Medical Treatment

Antibacterial therapy is indicated when UTI exists and is responsible for symptoms. Bacteria are almost invariably present in the urine of these patients. We do not think that asymptomatic bacteriuria must be submitted to any form of treatment as long as the colony count (Kass) does not exceed 1 million germs.

On the contrary, however, if the child is symptomatic and/or the colony count higher than 10 million suppressive low-dose long-term chemotherapy

Table 9.1

	Detrusor	Sphincter
Alpha-stimulation	+	+
ex: Etilephrine		−
Beta-stimulation	−	+
ex: Isuprel		−
Alpha-block	−	−
ex: Dybeniline		
Beta-block	−	+
ex: Propanolol		−
Cholinergic	+	+
ex: Urecholine		−
Anticholinergic	−	?
ex: Ditropan		
Others	−	+
ex: Tofranyl-Valium		

is indicated with usual anti-bacterial agents such as trimethoprim/sulfa-metho/azole (Bactrim), nitropoline (Nibiol), nitrofurantoin (Furadoine) with one half or one third of the usual dose, 5 days per week, alternatively. However, the best treatment of UTI is regular and complete bladder emptying.

Pharmacological agents are used for modifying bladder and sphincter tone. Almost all sympatheticometics and parasympatheticomimetics and/ or anticholinergic agents have been claimed to give excellent results in all possible bladder conditions (Table 9.1). It is our impression that only anticholinergic medication such as bethanecholchloride (Urecholine 1 to 2 pills) or oxybutyninechlorure (Ditropan 1 to 2 pills by day), have a valuable effect in decreasing bladder hypertonicity. Some added effects can be achieved with imipramine (Tofranil) or even diazapam (Valium). These drugs usually have an effect on the intestinal peristalsis and create constipation in most children.

Physiotherapy

It is often difficult to preserve normal anatomic conditions with a simple Crede maneuver repeated 5 to 6 times daily by the mother. We have not succeeded for longer than 18 months to 2 years. Moreover, this method is dangerous in the presence of vesicoureteral reflux by transmitting to the kidney the high pressure always necessary to force the sphincter resistance, the level of which is elevated by abdominal pressure in case of vesicosphincteric dyssynergia. Problems are more or less the same with Valsalva's procedure.

Clean intermittent catheterisation (CIC) must be considered as the major advance in the treatment of neurologic vesical dysfunction in the past 10 years. Introduced by Lapides (3) in adults, then by Lyon (4) in infants, CIC must be performed by the patient himself, or the parents, and must be considered as one of the most difficult tasks of multidisciplinary clinics. It requires more or less a lifetime involvement and may permanently alter the family's daily schedule. It can be started at any age, even in the young boy if necessary, and might be extremely efficient for control of UTI, distention and reflux. However, if the child's condition is stable, CIC is not initiated until school age, when social acceptance becomes a major factor. In our experience self catheterization might be initiated between ages 8 and 10, rarely earlier. Continence, however, will rarely be achieved without the help of pharmacology.

Clean intermittent catheterization must be performed every 3 hours, which means 5 to 6 times daily. It is not routinely associated with antibacterial therapy, but is almost invariably associated with propantheline bromide (Pro-Banthine 7.5 to 15 mg tid) or oxybutynin chloride (Ditropan 2.5 to 5 mg tid), both of which act to lower bladder pressure. Their subministration is sometimes associated with an attempt to increase bladder outlet resistance with ephedrine (10 to 25 mg) or imipramine (Tofranil).

With this program ⅔ of the patients respond favorably by achieving continence, avoiding UTI and preserving upper and lower tracts from deterioration. However, problems can occur related to deterioration of the system by various mechanisms such as urethral irritation or "fausse route" in boys, and difficulties in reaching the perineum in obese and paraplegic girls. Great progress has been made by permitting CIC through a continent cystostomy by using the appendix or ureter, after closure of the bladder neck (Fig. 9.9) (6).

Clean intermittent catheterization has also permitted the reintroduction of cystoenteroplasty for bladder augmentation, which had been abandoned in the past because of the difficulty of complete emptying.

Surgery

Most endoscopic sphincterotomies, bladder neck resections, divulsions, and urethral dilatations are no longer performed (except in very few selected cases) because they usually create a nonreversible situation of complete incontinence to then be treated by an artificial sphincter.

The surgical approach to these patients is actually directed toward vesicoureteral reflux, bladder augmentation, urinary diversion, and artificial sphincter.

Vesicoureteral Reflux

Our first impression has been that most of the patients with low-grade reflux can be successfully managed with CIC and pharmacology. With time, however, we have changed our policy to a more aggressive approach made possible by the excellent results of the Cohen cross-trigonal reim-

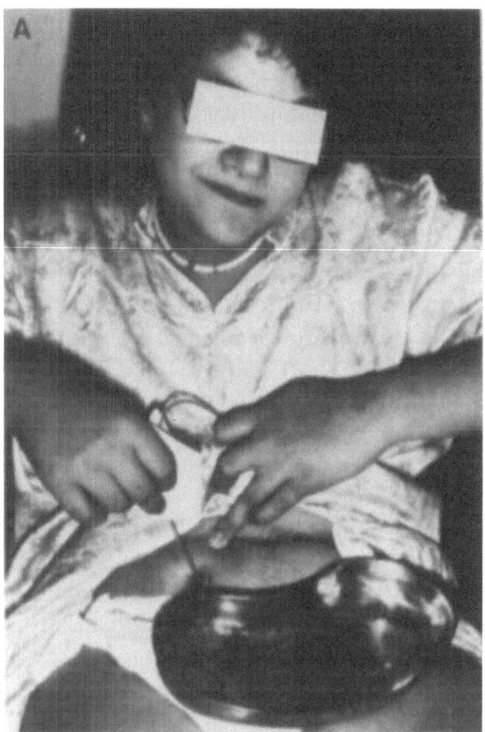

Figure 9.9. A Self-catheterization through an appendico-vesicostomy in an obese and paraplegic girl. B Normal upper urinary tract and close bladder neck with the catheter in the appendix.

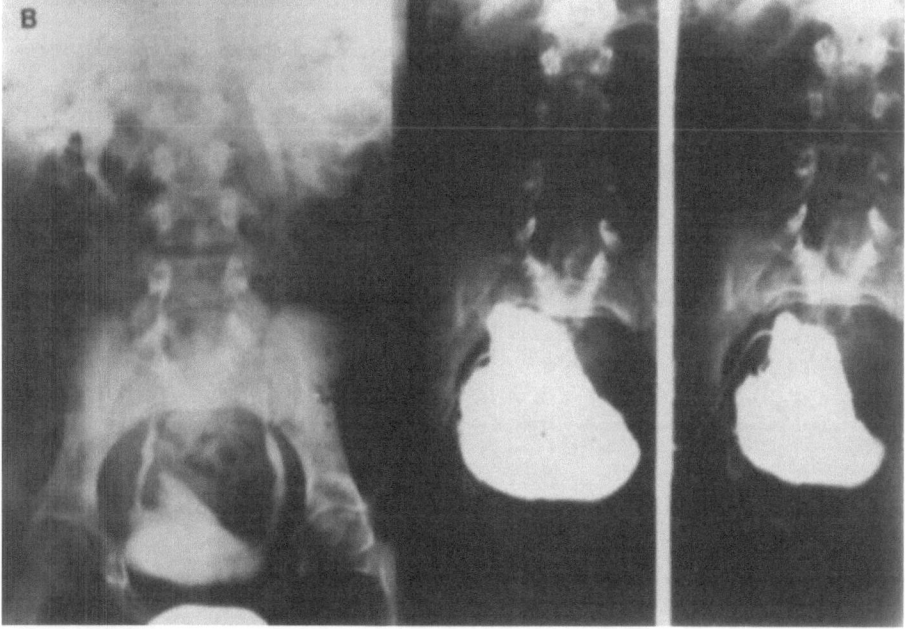

plantation of ureters, which we have performed in patients with both low-grade and high-grade reflux.

It was previously felt that severe reflux was better managed by urinary diversion. Now, most children with grades 4 or 5 reflux can receive implantation successfully. Reimplantation must be performed when failure of CIC is exemplified by persistent or increasing reflux, UTI or diminution of renal function based on isotopic renal studies and concentration ability (Fig. 9.10).

When the bladder is heavily trabeculated, however, although the ureters are anchored to the trigone, which usually has not deteriorated, results appear to be less favorable, especially in the adolescent age group. The exact mechanism of this bladder muscular hypertrophy is not perfectly clear, but is almost invariably associated with high outlet resistance, bladder hyperactivity, and hypertonicity.

If these conditions are under control before the anatomic deterioration is too far advanced, they can respond favorably to drug treatment (as previously shown). Antireflux surgery, together with CIC, can succeed in achieving continence and preserving the upper tract from deterioration.

Bladder augmentation muscular hypertrophy can often be associated with fibrotic involution of the bladder wall and will not respond to any sort of pharmacological treatment. In this case it might be of some interest

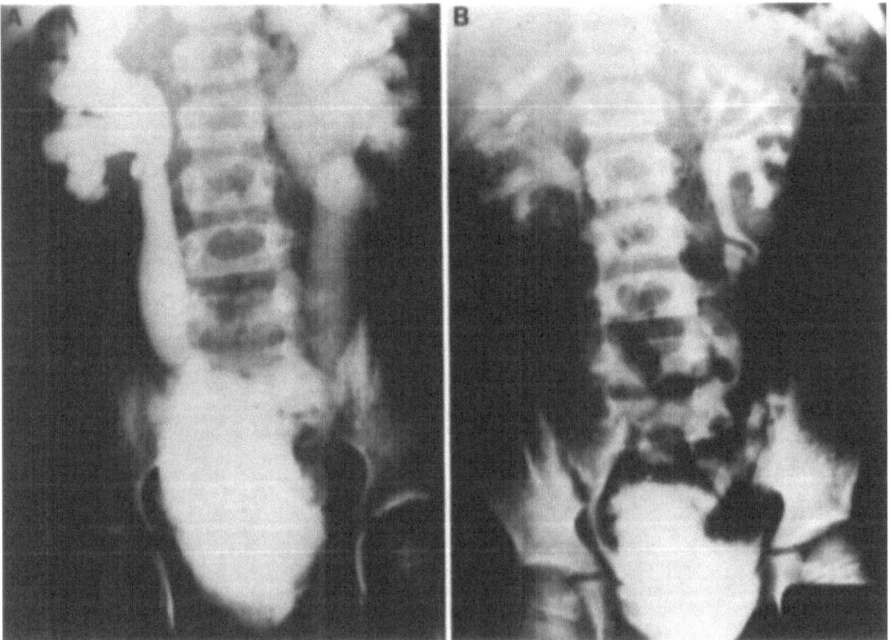

Figure 9.10. Pre- and postoperative upper urinary tract in a patient with massive stage 5 secondary reflux.

to increase bladder volume and to lower bladder pressure by bladder augmentation with cystoenteroplasty (Fig. 9.11). This usually transforms a high-pressure reservoir into a low compliance system. A simultaneous antireflux procedure can also be accomplished. However, these reservoirs are unable to achieve complete emptying and may have contraction of

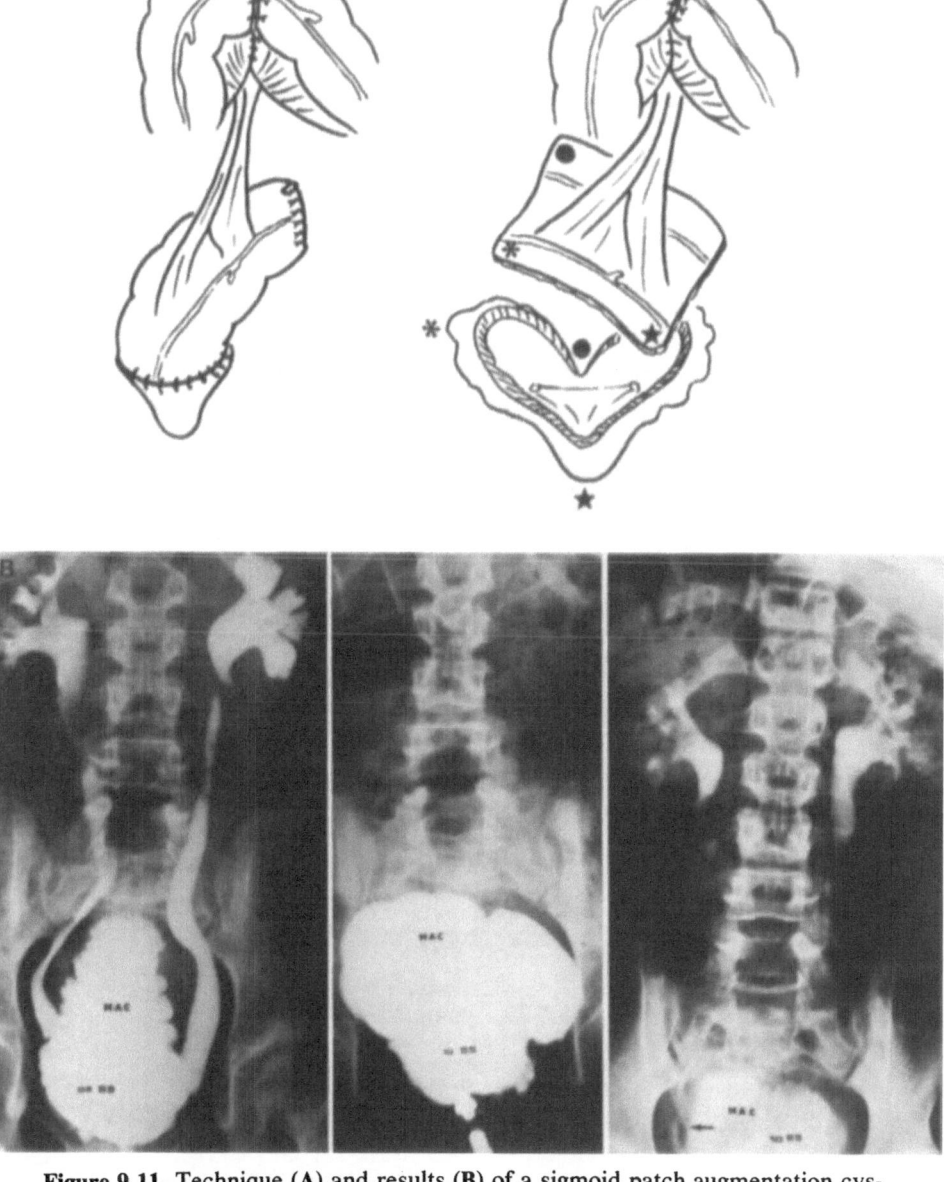

Figure 9.11. Technique **(A)** and results **(B)** of a sigmoid patch augmentation cystoenteroplasty.

their own, thus giving some leakage. They must then be used with CIC
and with an artificial sphincter system as well.

Diversion and Undiversion

The patients in whom continence is the most difficult problem to manage
are those who are either born with, or develop, severe upper tract changes
or significant bladder decompensation, or who suffer from brain damage.
In the past, these children were immediately subjected to permanent urinary diversion. At present, all attempts are directed toward keeping the
urinary tract internalized or, at most, performing a temporary, possibly
continent, diversion. Most patients in this particular group will benefit
from a temporary vesicostomy, either by the Blocksom technique (1,2)
or tubeless cystostomy (3). In our experience, closure is simple and anatomic conditions return to what they were previously.

Artificial Sphincter (Fig. 9.12)

The insertion of an artificial sphincter should be done only in extremely
critical cases. Further, the AMS 800 sphincter should be placed only in
children who have strong motivation, intelligent understanding to operate
the sphincter, smooth bladder with a large capacity, and a normal upper

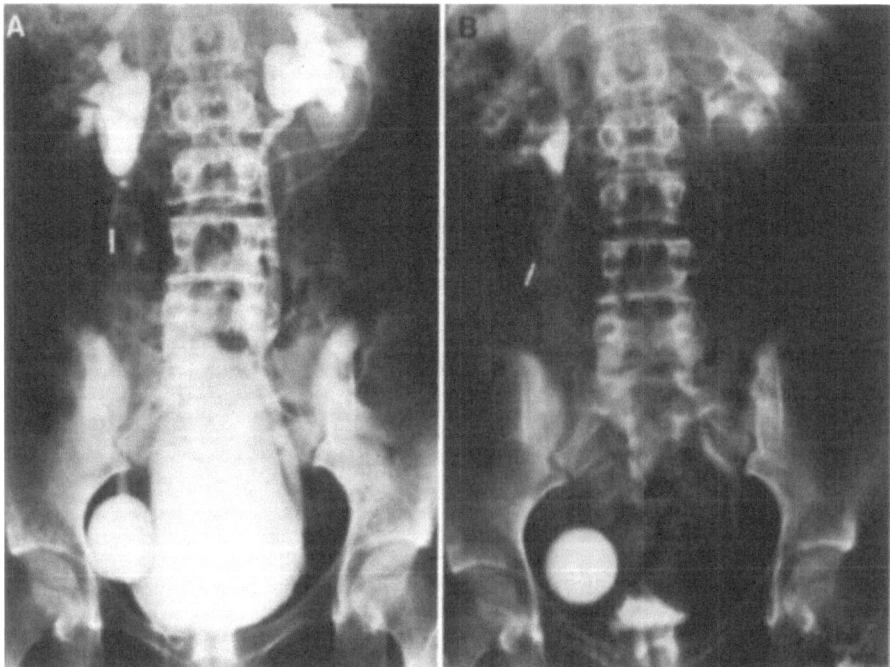

Figure 9.12. Artificial sphincter in place before (**A**) and after (**B**) micturition.

urinary tract. They must also learn to empty perfectly the bladder, either by abdominal pressure or CIC, on a routine basis, otherwise compliance will slowly decrease, giving less good quality of life with time.

If a baby is born with a complete neurologic lesion, he usually needs only a yearly renal sonogram and periodic checking of residual urine (Figs. 9.13, 9.14). The lower urinary tract is generally unobstructed and he is at low risk for deterioration (SR 20 cm of water).

Programs to achieve better social life and continence should not start before school age. Conversely, if a child has an abnormal intravenous pyelogram or a UTI is recommended, a repeat voiding cystouretrography to look for both obstruction (SR = 40 cm) and reflux, and an operation must be performed to avoid any deterioration, secondary to distention, hypertonicity, or reflux. In the very young, the best solution remains a temporary, tubeless cystostomy (no prolapse), easily performed and closed, when the child himself, asks for it. Without severe brain damage, most of these patients might reach adulthood with normal upper urinary tract, good bladder capacity, and bladder continence. This is one of the major successes of modern pediatric urology.

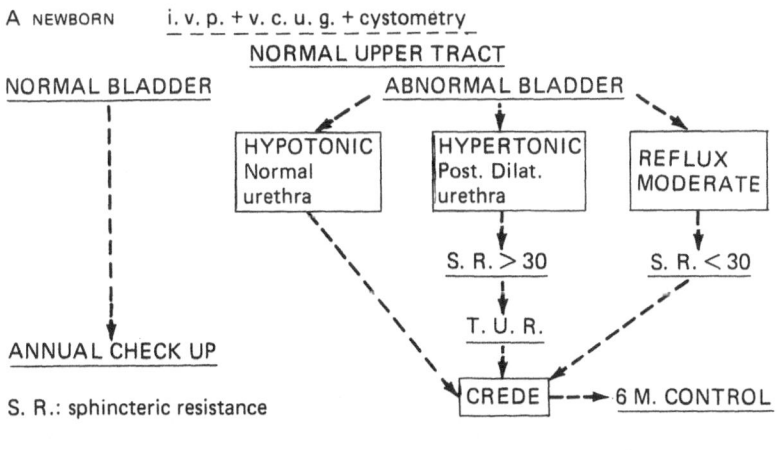

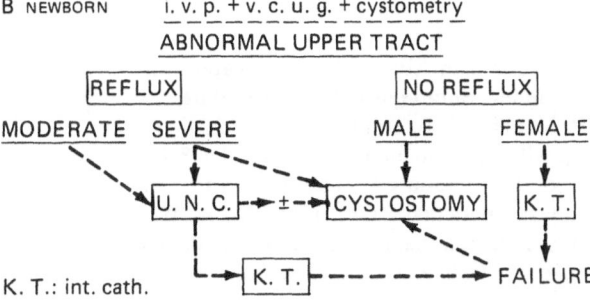

Figure 9.13. Therapeutic approach to MMC in the newborn period.

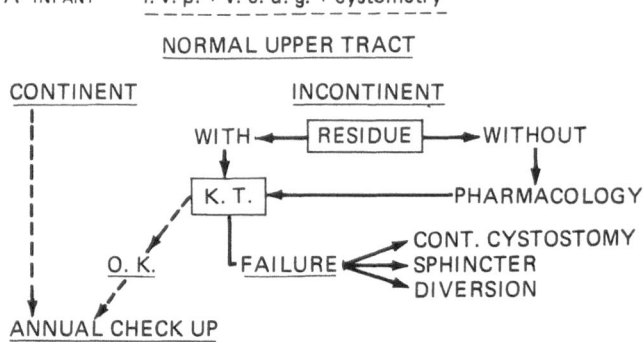

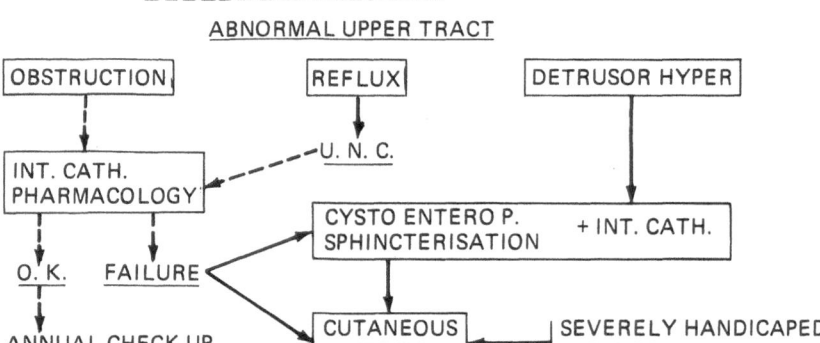

Figure 9.14. Therapeutic approach to MMC in infancy.

References

1. Duckett JWJ, Raezer DM: Neuromuscular dysfunction of urinary bladder, in Kelalis PP, King LR (eds): Clinical pediatric urology. Philadelphia: Saunders, 1976.
2. Duckett JW Jr: Cutaneous vesicostomy in childhood: the Blocksom technique. Urol Clin North Am 1:485, 1974.
3. Lapides J, Friend CR, Ajemian EP, et al.: Denervation supersensitivity as a test for neurogenic bladder. Surg Gynecol 114:241, 1962.
4. Lyon RP, Scott MP, Marshall S: Intermittent catheterization rather than urinary diversion in children with myelomeningocele. J Urol 113:409, 1975.
5. McGuire EJ, Woodside JR, Borden TA, et al: Prognostic value of urodynamics testing in myelodysplastic patients. J Urol 126:205–209, 1981.
6. Mitrofanoff P: Cystostomie continente trans-appendiculaire dans le traitement des vessies neurologiques. Chir Pédiat 21:97, 1980.

Index

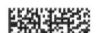